COSMETIC
DERMATOLOGIC SURGERY

Cosmetic Dermatologic Surgery

Samuel J. Stegman, M.D.
Associate Clinical Professor in Dermatology

Theodore A. Tromovitch, M.D.
Clinical Professor in Dermatology

University of California, San Francisco, School of Medicine
San Francisco, California

YEAR BOOK MEDICAL PUBLISHERS, INC.
CHICAGO • LONDON

Library of Congress Cataloging in Publication Data

Stegman, Samuel J.
    Cosmetic dermatologic surgery.

    Includes index.
    1. Skin—Surgery.   2. Surgery, Plastic.
I. Tromovitch, Theodore A.   II. Title.   [DNLM:
1. Surgery, Plastic.   WO 600 S817c]
RD520.S733   1983   617′.4770592   83-6784
ISBN 0-8151-8169-8

DEDICATION

To our parents,
MRS. JOHN STEGMAN
and MR. *and* MRS. ALBERT TROMOVITCH

Contents

Preface

DR. EUGENE TARDY, a renowned facial plastic surgeon of Chicago, Illinois, has stated in presentations to physicians that the greatest amount of cosmetic surgery is done by dermatologists. He was referring mostly to the many cosmetic procedures such as hair transplants, dermabrasion, and chemical peels that have been the purview of this specialty for many years. He is also referring to the multitudes of small blemishes and lesions that are routinely treated by dermatologists. The management of telangiectasias, nevi, hypertrophic scars and keloids, and many other benign lesions are often not thought of as cosmetic surgery. But indeed they are.

Although there are some chapters in this book about procedures that are not routinely performed by all dermatologists, all dermatologists will be surprised by the number of procedures that are cosmetic and are routinely performed in the dermatology office. We believe that it would be valuable for our colleagues to have the scope of cosmetic dermatologic surgery available in one small, usable text. All of the procedures discussed can be performed in the office under local anesthesia.

We owe a great debt of thanks to Dr. Ralph Luikart for his contribution of the chapter on face lifts. Doctor Luikart has been a forerunner of dermatologic cosmetic surgery for many years. It is only of late that the rest of us are realizing his foresight and are joining him in his definition of the scope of our specialty.

We owe special thanks to Susan Cristian for her chapter on cosmetic consultation. Her services and those of her profession are extremely valuable to any physician performing cosmetic surgery and for any physician concerned about those conditions for which cosmetic camouflage is the treatment of choice.

This text, in a large part, was the product of our faithful and tireless secretary, Marian Ward, and the special creative skills of our medical illustrator, Susan Wong. We owe these ladies a tremendous debt.

Also, a special thanks to our photographer, Sara Douglas, whose excellent photography added to the visual quality and educational potential of these texts.

SAMUEL J. STEGMAN, M.D.

THEODORE A. TROMOVITCH, M.D.

COSMETIC
DERMATOLOGIC SURGERY

Color Plates

PLATE I

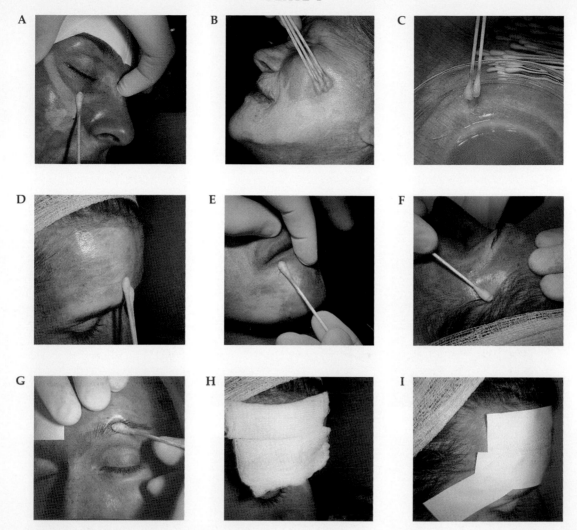

Plate I.—Technique for phenol peels. **A,** use of one cotton-tipped applicator around eyelids. **B,** use of three applicators for broad areas. **C,** cotton tips are used to stir the peel mixture and then are pressed dry against the side of the dish. **D,** appearance of frosting when using Baker's formula. **E,** removal of lip wrinkles re-quires that the agent be taken beyond the vermilion border. **F** and **G,** around hair-bearing areas the agent is carried into the hairline. **H,** placement of cool compress over the treated area. **I,** placement of tape used in the peel.

PLATE II

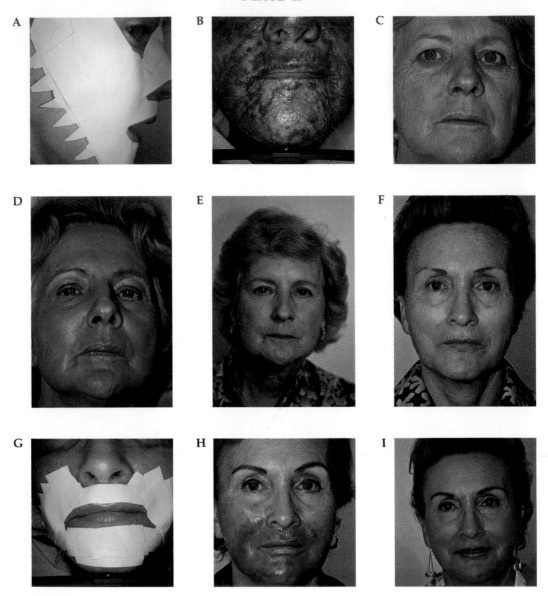

Plate II.—Technique for phenol peels (cont.). **A,** application of tape mask in a saw-tooth-like fashion at the mandible margin. **B,** appearance after removal of tape mask. **C,** A 60-year-old patient before a full-face Baker's formula occluded peel; **D,** three months after the surgery; and **E,** four years after the surgery. She also had an upper lid blepharoplasty. **F–H,** This 55-year-old woman had more severe aging changes of the lower one-third of her face, so a Baker's formula phenol peel with occlusion was performed on the perioral cosmetic unit with blending onto the cheeks where an occluded Baker's formula phenol peel was carried to the level of the temples and the lower eyelids. **I,** patient six months after surgery with her normal makeup.

PLATE III

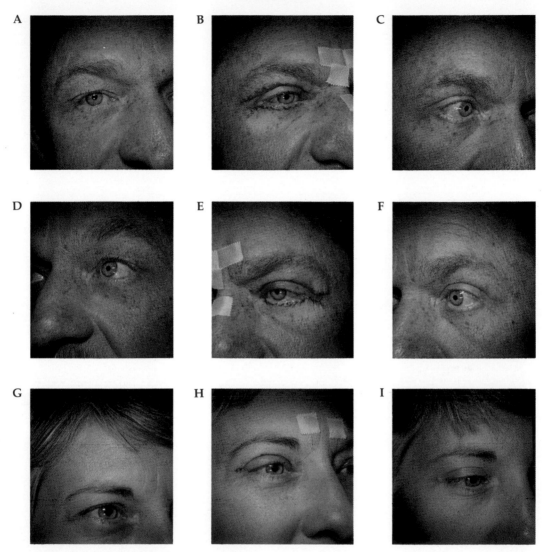

Plate III.—Blepharoplasty and lipectomy. **A,** appearance of right eye prior to surgery. **B,** appearance immediately postsurgery. **C,** appearance one month postsurgery. **D,** appearance of left eye of same patient as **A** before surgery. **E,** appearance immediately postsurgery. **F,** appearance one month postsurgery. **G,** appearance of right eye before surgery. **H,** appearance immediately postsurgery. **I,** appearance one month postsurgery.

PLATE IV

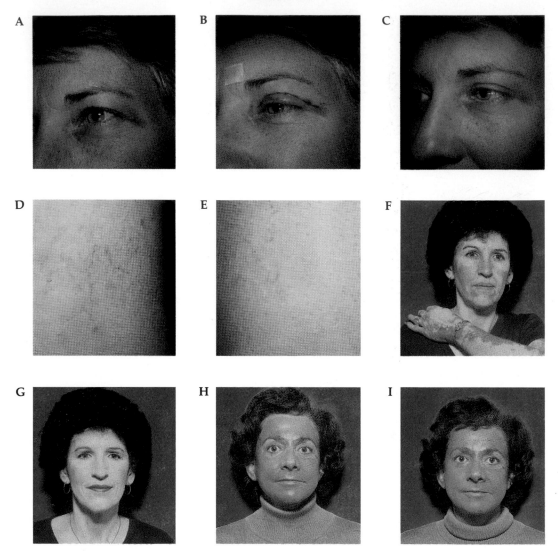

Plate IV.—**A, B, C,** Blepharoplasty and lipectomy, same patient as in Plate III, **G, H, I. A,** appearance of left eye before surgery. **B,** appearance immediately postsurgery. **C,** appearance one month postsurgery. **D,** telangiectasia of the legs before treatment. **E,** appearance of patient in **D** and treatment was complete. **F,** 45-year-old female suffering from minor hypopigmentation. **G,** patient in **F** after coverage with *L.E. Velvet Film* and makeup. **H,** appearance of a patent 14 days after a chemical peel. **I,** appearance of patient in H after an application of a sunscreen preparation and a muting cream.

1 / General Principles of Office Cosmetic Surgery

THE GOAL

THE PATIENT'S REAL GOAL in wanting a cosmetic procedure is subjective and sometimes occult—even to the patient. Failure to recognize this fact can lead to patient dissatisfaction and prolonged anxiety for the physician. On the other hand, if he realizes that the patient visit for a cosmetic procedure is much different from a visit for a physical ailment or medical examination, the physician can smoothly and efficiently change his approach and incorporate the simple and subtle differences needed to deal with a cosmetic problem.

The results of cosmetic surgery are subjective. Consequently, excising, changing, or correcting the obvious does not necessarily lead to success. It is essential to discover the true motivation and what the patient hopes to achieve physically, remembering that the desire to be more sexually attractive or to feel better psychologically about one's physical appearance sometimes is the true reason for wanting the physical change. Thus, an office consultation for cosmetic surgery can be more personal than any other type of visit. Granted, illness is a personal event; however, most people view illness as an externally caused problem. On the other hand, the patient usually considers the cosmetic procedure extremely personal, sometimes embarrassing or even inordinately foolish. The physician should approach each cosmetic patient as one with a delicate and personal problem, thus avoiding the unproductive and unpleasant mistake of confronting the patient too directly and abruptly.

Feelings of guilt and vanity often are present in varying degrees. These emotions cloud direct communication. The glib and sophisticated patient easily can recite many "right" reasons for requesting a certain procedure, but how many tell or even know the true reasons? On the other hand, the less verbally communicative patient may only point and shrug. In each situation one must ferret out the needed information. All of this extra work *before* a cosmetic procedure can prevent hours of anguish for the patient and the physician *afterward*.

SCHEDULING COSMETIC CONSULTATIONS

A cosmetic consultation must not be hurried or even seem to be hurried. Most patients have not had a cosmetic surgery consultation, and the whole procedure is new to them. Even for the simplest problem, allow a little extra time to communicate with patients about what they want you to do and what you plan to do.

Beware of "While I've got you here, Doctor" consultations. Many patients are too embarrassed to schedule a cosmetic consultation and will ask you about something that is extremely important to them at the close of a regular or fabricated regular visit. Listen closely and be ready to deal with such questions appropriately. If you can answer simply within the time of the office visit, sit down and talk. However, if the problem is complicated, mention a few points that might have to be discussed at length and schedule an appropriate consultation.

For most office cosmetic procedures, a patient will be scheduled among routine office visits. It is a luxury for some physicians to have cosmetic afternoons or an entire practice limited to cosmetic problems. For most of us, minor cosmetic problems are just one part of our practice, and these patients are seen in line with our other patients. If the office assistants, particularly the booking assistant, and the physician all are aware of the need to change style for a cosmetic visit, seeing these patients with other medical patients can be accomplished appropriately and smoothly.

Follow-up visits for cosmetic patients are just as important as initial visits and often are just as time-consuming. Failure to recover from a medical illness after a single office visit does not surprise most patients. They will accept the need for revisits, plan to pay for them, and become frustrated with their own illness rather than with the physician. On the other hand, a cosmetic procedure often is perceived as a one-time-only event that will completely heal or be resolved within an allotted period. If the goal has not been achieved when and as expected, frustration and dissatisfaction often are directed toward the physician. The dissatisfaction becomes a barrier. Anxieties arise, communication fails, and what could have been an acceptable or successful office visit becomes uncomfortable for both patient and physician.

Although the temptation is strong not to reschedule a troublesome patient, it is exactly the wrong thing to do. If the patient needs more support, schedule appointments more frequently and allot more time for each visit. It is a good idea never to dismiss completely a postcosmetic surgery patient. Always leave the door open for time to come back whenever the patient feels the need or always offer consultation from a colleague as a second opinion for further remedial procedure(s).

THE CONSULTATION

The cosmetic surgery consultation includes the following assessments: (1) that sufficient physical alteration has occurred to warrant treatment, (2) that the patient has a good psychological outlook, (3) that the proposed treatment will sufficiently correct the defect(s) presented by the patient, and (4) that the physician knows as accurately as possible how the patient visualizes the defect and what improvement he or she expects.

Studies have shown that, in general, the best patient is a person who has a significant cosmetic defect, has had it for a long time, is requesting the cosmetic procedure because of a desire to present a better image, and is otherwise reasonably well balanced psychologically. This patient profile produces the happiest patient after cosmetic surgery regardless of the type of procedure.

For a cosmetic consultation, the first thing we do is to give the patient a hand mirror and a cotton applicator stick. We ask that the wooden end of the Q-tip be used as a pointer to indicate exactly where the problem is. Do not be fooled by the question "Well, don't you see the problem, Doctor?" Too many times we have seen a problem, but it was not the one that concerned the patient. Such a visit starts with an awkward moment. Gently, we encourage the patient to tell us what he or she sees as bothersome. This is true whether the problem is only a mole or the entire complexion. We also ask the patient to describe why the lesions are a problem. We try to disarm the patient by saying, ''We're playing a little game now, but it helps us to understand how we can help you in the best possible way.'' This sentence usually allows the patient to open up and to explain the problem freely. For a medical office visit, we all know that history is quite important. The history in a cosmetic visit consists of the patient's telling you what the problem is and why it is bothersome, how treatment may improve appearance, and what specific results are expected. It cannot be overemphasized how important it is for the patient to do as much of the talking as possible during the first part of a cosmetic consultation.

Next, examine the patient. Examine the entire face and the area under question, as well as hair and nails, and briefly examine other medical problems. At this point there is an opportunity that you may not have at any other time. You can bring up other cosmetic problems that are amenable to treatment that the patient did not mention. Usually we say, ''Since you ask about matters concerning your appearance, maybe you will let me tell you about some other features that may be improved.'' This statement almost always is successful in letting us point out to the patient, without any offense, something else that might be treated. The response will quickly signal the patient's feelings. An extremely large, unsightly mole that you have pointed out often will be dismissed with the comment '' . . .well, I've always had that as a family trait.'' Then you know to stay away from that mole because to take it off would cause you trouble later. On the other hand, if you point out sebaceous hyperplasia, redundant eyelid tissue, or an unsightly scar that could be revised and tell the patient that these blemishes are treatable, the patient will be encouraged by your thoroughness and often will be receptive to your suggestions.

At this point of the consultation, it is time for the physician to become the main speaker. The physician first should address the problem that the patient asked about. If he has received permission, either directly or indirectly, to discuss other problems, they can be included in the discussion. If not, he should restrict his discussion to the area that the patient described. The physician should have in mind a complete and thorough explanation that he delivers to each patient concerning each cosmetic procedure. This can be complemented with printed handout material, photograph albums, slide-tape patient education programs, videotape education programs, etc. However, nothing will replace the time that the physician spends with the patient explaining the procedure. It should be an orderly explanation, including the procedure with all details, the morbidity, the prognosis, the risks, and the side effects. How detailed and how much of each of these subjects is discussed varies with the patient, the procedure, and the amount of additional material presented at the time of the consultation. If complications develop, their management is greatly facilitated if the physician can say, ''Well, Mrs. Smith, you developed one of those problems that we told you about when we first discussed your surgery. Let's see what we can do to help you with it.''

The single most important result of a cosmetic consultation is that the patient *understands* what you think will be the *result* of this procedure. Fulfilling this obligation is predicated on the fact that you are able to communicate with the patient and that he/she is receptive to the information. Both criteria are extremely complicated and difficult to fulfill.

There are five tasks that should be accomplished by the close of the cosmetic consultation. First, encourage the patient to delay making any decisions. Many patients have thought about the procedure that they are requesting. If the results of your consultation agree with their previous information, they will be ready to schedule the surgery. This is acceptable, but it is important for you to be sure that these patients have done all of their homework previously and really understand the procedure. Usually, some amount of time to consider what you have told them is desirable. We always recommend that patients call us for further information whenever questions arise. Sometimes we offer them the names of other physicians for second opinions and other times we offer them another consultation in the office if more involved questions need to be discussed.

Second, we insist that before the day of the surgery patients understand all of the procedure and follow-up procedures. They should not come to the office on the day of the surgery with a long list of unanswered questions.

Third, for extensive cosmetic procedures, we require payment at the time the appointment is made. Payment in advance is beneficial to both the patient and the physician. It reduces the number of cancellations and insures a high rate of patient compliance. It is beneficial to the patients because it forces them to decide whether or not they want the procedure. Once they have paid for it, they usually have made a firm commitment and it is easier for them to go ahead. If they have not paid, they will allow themselves to worry, stall, debate, and agonize over the decision.

Fourth, the patient should understand that you cannot predict precisely the final outcome, only that you will strive for maximum improvement. Almost everyone doing cosmetic surgery has had a patient in whom little benefit was achieved as judged objectively but a great benefit was perceived by the patient, with significant change in life attitudes. Similarly, essentially perfect cosmetic results have resulted in a disappointed, angry, and lawsuit-threatening patient because the patient expected more than any cosmetic surgeon could deliver. Do not promise too much to the patient. It is better not to define specific results but to talk about improvement that may be obtained.

Fifth, it is important to document all of the information from the consultation. There are many good ways to document the information that the patient has received. *All* of them can be attacked by lawyers. *All* of them can be ignored by juries. There is no such thing as a perfect documentation of what the patient was told. However, the physician should demonstrate diligence, reasonable recording, and a sincere effort to tell the patient what can be expected for the problem. If a sincere documentation attempt has been made, the physician can rest assured that he has done his job. How society and the jousting of the adversary system later deal with his work is too unpredictable to waste more than an insurance premium on.

DAY OF SURGERY

See the patient before the administration of any preanesthetic agents. The patient should be greeted and the event established as a happy one. This is an important day in the patient's life; it should be a happy day and not one of inordinate fear. Some anxieties are normal, but they should be interpreted as the expectation of a happy event. In a brief visit with the patient, any final questions can be answered, a review of the day's expectations can be summarized, and photographs taken. Before any preanesthesia is given, the patient must be assured that the physician is on the premises, in good spirits, and ready to devote his entire attention and skills to that patient alone. The office should seem efficient and organized, and all other activities should give the impression that they now are being directed toward the patient. Following these simple steps can relieve anxiety far more than huge amounts of medication.

2 / Benign Facial Lesions

WHEN EXAMINING A PATIENT for any cosmetic procedure, look closely at all aspects of the skin of the face, neck, and other exposed areas. Many times an uneven appearance is not the result of any one lesion but the product of multiple lesions, such as telangiectasia, milia, nevi, lentigines, sebaceous hyperplasia, melasma, rosacea, seborrheic dermatitis, etc. It is not uncommon for patients to have many of these separate, benign entities. A well-done blepharoplasty, face peel, or dermabrasion alone still may leave the patient with distracting benign lesions that could have been handled simply before or in conjunction with other procedures.

There are patients who need not undergo a major cosmetic procedure but whose appearance can be improved greatly simply by treating the small benign lesions. Because these lesions are of slow onset and are recognized by the patient to be benign, just how unsightly and distracting they are often is not appreciated. Sometimes the physician may mention to the patient that such and such a distracting lesion is benign and is simple to treat in the office. It is risky, though; patients can be easily offended by such well-meaning statements. We never cease to be amazed at the lumps and bumps that patients can learn to tolerate.

TELANGIECTASIA

These small, linear superficial, ectatic vessels (Fig 2–1) often are mistakenly associated with excessive alcohol consumption. Often it is this false association that causes the patient to seek treatment. Although there may be some telangiectasias formed as part of acne rosacea, actinic damage, or prolonged use of high-potency corticosteroid creams on the face, most of the time the physician does not know the true etiology. The patient should be encouraged to seek treatment because a simple procedure will improve the overall ruddy appearance or will decrease easily noticed telangiectasias. Other than modifying the above-mentioned causes, there is no advice for patients as to how to prevent further development of these lesions. The patient needs to understand that treatment of existing lesions in no way affects the development of further lesions.

For telangiectasias on the face, the best treatment is electrodesiccation with a damped, high-voltage, low-amperage, bipolar current administered through an epilating needle (Fig 2–2). The bipolar current is preferable to the monopolar. However, many use the simple Birtcher hyfrecator because its frequent use in office surgery makes it readily available. For first-time treatment and simple telangiectasias, we routinely use the Birtcher hyfrecator. However, for recurrent or larger ones, we will use a bipolar instrument. The epilating needle is held on or just above the skin, over the telangiectasia. It is not necessary to try

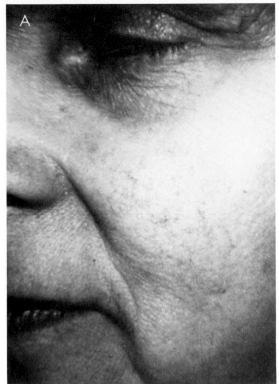

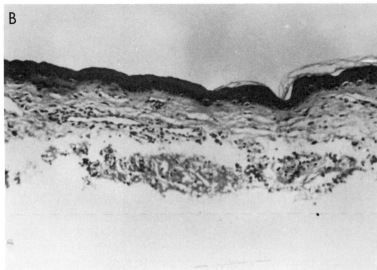

Fig 2–1.—Telangiectasia of the face. **A,** gross appearance. **B,** microscopic appearance.

Fig 2–2.—Technique of treatment for telangiectasia with an epilating needle.

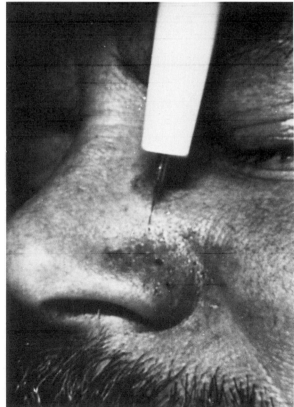

to probe or cannulate the tiny vessel. The current jumps to the surface and through the skin to the more conductive blood in the vessel. The current usually will travel some distance through the vessel itself. If many lesions are to be treated, the setting on the instrument may require adjustment during the treatment because of changes in efficiency of the machine or the current in the office building, which changes with the demands made by elevators and other electric equipment.

We try to explain briefly to the patients what is going to happen, but tell them that they will be able to relax best after we have demonstrated that the procedure really is not very painful. We try to give them one or two pulses of the current so that they realize that the discomfort is easily tolerated. We try to start on the middle to lower cheeks, working toward the upper cheeks and the eyes and then across the nose. We save the nose and the area around the eyes for last because they are more sensitive to pain and also because electrodesiccation near the columella or on the nasal alae tends to elicit tear responses and sneezing reflexes.

The mechanism of action is that the current passing through the tiny vessel walls irritates the walls. They become edematous and eventually swell shut. Many of them remain shut and do not recanalize, but some will, and the patient must realize that some will recur. In the sebaceous skin around the nasal alae, the treatment of the vessels often will leave a tiny depressed trough. The patients should be forewarned that for the vessels in this area, they will be trading the sometimes quite obvious purple telangiectasias for the risk of having a small trough or valley, which, to our eyes, is more cosmetically acceptable. Sometimes there is a small mark at the site where the needle was held over the skin. On the face, this almost always heals without any blemish. If blemishes do develop in the occasional patient, the only prevention might be to use a less-intense current.

On the face, we will treat as many telangiectasias in one sitting as the patients will tolerate. Often, however, they prefer to have ten to 20 done per visit and then return for touch-ups. If the vessels are extremely large, it is less likely that they will swell shut and stay uncanalized. For the extremely large telangiectasia, it is not necessarily wise to use a higher current, since this increases the possibility of scarring at the site where the needle was held over the skin. For the very large facial telangiectasias, the only other modality is a dermabrasion. Lasers have been used for telangiectasias, but are reported to leave a circular or linear white scar, which often is not a fair trade-off for the telangiectasia. Some patients find this white mark more objectionable than a telangiectasia.

Telangiectasias are treated successfully with electrocoagulation anywhere on the face, upper anterior neck, and anterior chest. We also treat telangiectasias on the forearms and the backs of the hands, but results are not always permanent. As a general rule, the farther one strays from the face the greater the incidence of the small pinpoint scar at the site where the needle was held over the skin. For reasons we do not understand, telangiectasias on the lower extremities do not respond nearly as well. Although we know of good office cosmetic surgeons who will treat telangiectasias on the thigh and calf with electrocoagulation, we have not been happy with the results ourselves. There seems to be a high incidence of the small pinpoint scars developing along a track as the physician moves the needle along the surface of the large vessels. We believe that telangiectasias of the lower extremities are best treated by injection, which will be discussed in chapter 15.

In our hands, the bipolar current is not necessary for most telangiectasias, particularly on the face. However, for a large spider nevus (nevus arachnoideus) with a large central pulsating arteriol that has not responded to treatment with monopolar current, the bipolar current usually is necessary.

Because the telangiectasia will constrict with epinephrine, if local anesthesia is to be tried, it should be done without epinephrine. However, we usually can obtain patient cooperation and not use any anesthesia at all.

SPIDER NEVI

When treating a spider nevus (Fig 2–3,A), it is wise to advise the patient that he will be exchanging this large red blemish for what we hope will be a small, unnoticeable scar. The treatment is electrocoagulation (Fig 2–3,B). Sometimes

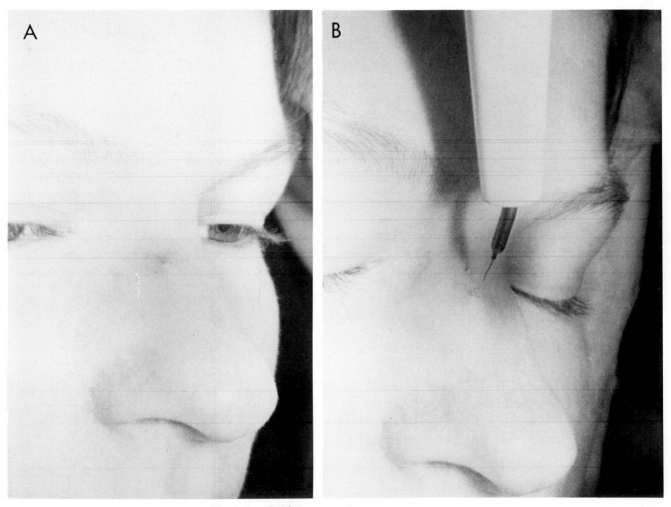

Fig 2–3.—Spider nevus. **A,** gross appearance.
B, treatment by electrocoagulation.

the lesions do not scar, but since occasionally they do, it is wise to have warned the patient. If a spider nevus recurs after what was believed to be adequate treatment with a bipolar current instrument, it may be necessary to excise the central vessel and the surrounding exuberant tissue with a punch excision technique.

Multiple spider nevi occasionally develop with liver disease and in the normal course of some pregnancies. Often the lesions fade after parturition. On the patient with liver disease there are so many lesions that the treatment for this simple condition probably is not practical, since the other manifestations of the liver disease are far more critical. Occasionally, however, a patient will request treatment of a spider nevus on an exposed area, and these nevi should respond to electrocoagulation as successfully as those not caused by obvious liver disease.

MILIA

Milia are inclusion cysts, usually 0.5–2.9 mm in diameter and commonly found on the face (Fig 2–4) and neck area. They appear after dermabrasion, face peel, and along suture lines, but these posttreatment milia usually have their onset two to three weeks after the surgery and last up to six months. Often they are self-limiting. Clinically, it is difficult to distinguish between closed comedones of acne and milia.

The treatment for milia is to unroof and drain them. Standard incision and drainage with a #11 scalpel Bard-Parker blade is an acceptable method, although we find it cumbersome. We use a Hagedorn needle and try to hold the milia steady, either by pinching it between the thumb and index finger or by holding the skin taut with three-finger pressure around it. The thin skin above milia is incised and the small amount of creamy material or inspissated core is

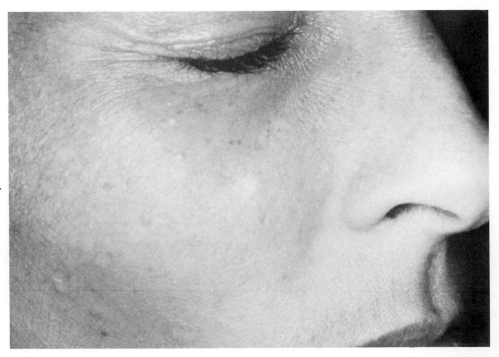

Fig 2–4.—Milia (inclusion cysts).

extruded. If possible, try to recover the small epithelial sac with the milia. Of late, we have been using hot cautery. The hot cautery fine-point tip is heated to just below red heat and tapped slightly on the thin skin on top of the milia. This is almost painless, or only slightly painful, and leads to drainage of the milia, with later drying and extrusion of the sac. These generally heal without scarring. Again, the patients are encouraged to allow the physician to treat one or two so that they will realize that the procedure does not hurt a great deal. After that, many can be done. With a cooperative patient, it is possible to do 30–60 of these milia per minute. They heal within just a few days.

The only disadvantage of using hot cautery is that the patient realizes that a hot instrument is being used, and if there is any blemish left in the area, it is difficult to convince the patient that the blemish is not the result of a severe burn.

Some physicians like to use a Birtcher hyfrecator on a very low setting, with the epilating needle, to electrodesiccate the milia. This also is quite acceptable and a quick way to treat these lesions. For the masses of milia that may form after dermabrasion or chemical peel, the patient can be simply reassured that they will clear spontaneously. However, for a few occasional milia it is a simple and rewarding treatment.

INTRADERMAL NEVI (MOLES)

It may seem unwarranted to discuss moles in a book on cosmetic surgery, but actually the subject matter is appropriate. These days only rarely is a mole considered a "beauty mark." Usually, individual moles and certainly multiple moles detract from the patient's appearance. The natural history of a mole can include pedunculation or becoming sessile. If either of these normal maturation patterns ensues, the patient can look warty, which carries the connotation of an aged, unkempt appearance. If the mole is deeply pigmented, sometimes its appearance is alarming; this, too, detracts from the cosmetic appeal.

Generally, patients will come to the office specifically for removal of a mole; and in these cases, it is a simple matter. However, if other cosmetic procedures are planned and a mole is near a surgical site, the surgeon can offer the patient the option of having it treated during or before the cosmetic surgery. At times, the patients will have forgotten about the mole because they have become so accustomed to it. They are surprised when you remind them how much it detracts from their cosmetic beauty. As mentioned previously, the appropriate time to mention that the moles are unsightly is when the patient is consulting the physician for other cosmetic problems.

Most intradermal nevi are benign and can be removed easily at the time of surgery. However, it is absolutely essential that the tissue removed be submitted for histopathologic examination. Each mole removed should be specifically numbered, or several moles can be color coded and placed within the same specimen bottle. Generally there is no reason to do a frozen section, and most melanotic lesions are best read with paraffin preparation.

We prefer the shave technique for simple intradermal nevi or for compound nevi. The shave technique is the simplest to perform, the least likely to leave an unsightly scar, and the postoperative care is negligible. However, there can be some spotty repigmentation at the site of the shave excision. For most patients, removal of the elevated portion of the mole is adequate, but if the patient insists that there be no residual color, performing complete excision with suture closure is necessary. It is important to realize that even exophytic non-pigmented nevi often will leave a pigmented macule after shave excision. We try to convince patients that shave excision usually is indicated, and we tell them that the lump will be gone, usually the color will be gone, and that the method provides an adequate specimen for histopathology. We advise them that if the residual pigmentary changes will be troublesome to them, a complete excision and closure will be necessary.

Healing after a shave excision generally is excellent on the face, scalp, and neck. However, there is a disturbingly high incidence of hypertrophic scarring from shave techniques on the anterior chest, the deltoid area, and the upper one-third of the back. Unfortunately, it is these areas in which a hypertrophic scar is bothersome if women want to wear low-cut clothing. To exchange a mole for a hypertrophic scar often is not a rewarding exercise. If the patient fully understands the chance of having a hypertrophic scar and is willing to accept the risk, the physician can comply. With excision and suture closure there always is the risk of a larger hypertrophic scar developing. This can lead to untold anguish if the patient does not fully understand the unsightliness and the risks of developing hypertrophic scarring.

If there are long, dark hairs protruding from the mole, remind the patient that these will regrow after the mole has been shaved. If the hairs are a problem, they can be treated by electric epilation. It is important that the patient understand this possibility and does not expect the hair to be gone after the shave technique.

Any mole can be excised completely, and, of course, suspicious moles should be excised with normal margins ranging from 2.0 to 5.0 mm.

We suggest that the physician not press the patient too hard to have moles removed if a simple suggestion does not lead the patient to consent. A patient who has any type of problem, real or imagined, after a mole is removed at the suggestion of the physician can cause a great deal of anguish for the physician. The patient returning two months after a simple mole shave excision with a hypertrophic or pigmented scar always will want to know why the physician insisted that it be removed and complain about the "terrible scar that looks worse than the mole ever did."

The technique for shave excision of a mole varies with the shape of the base of the mole. If it is a sessile or pedunculated mole, a tiny amount of lidocaine (Xylocaine) with epinephrine will make a bleb at the base, and then scissors can be used simply to excise the pedicle. A small drop of Monsel's solution or aluminum chloride is adequate for hemostasis. If the mole has a flat base, after local anesthesia, which tends to elevate the mole (Fig 2–5,A), the skin is pulled taut with three-finger tension (Fig 2–5,B) or with tension from an assistant and is carefully incised at the exact junction between the mole tissue and the normal skin. We like to use $2\times$ magnification through a head-magnifying hood to be able to observe carefully that junction. Using the scalpel, not in bold strokes but in repeated, small, sweeping strokes, we gradually "feel" our way across the base of the mole. If the assistant sponges and the physician uses his other hand to lift up the mole with the forceps, he can observe the mole and skin interface and cut just below it. This allows the mole to be chipped out with only a little normal skin excised at the same time.

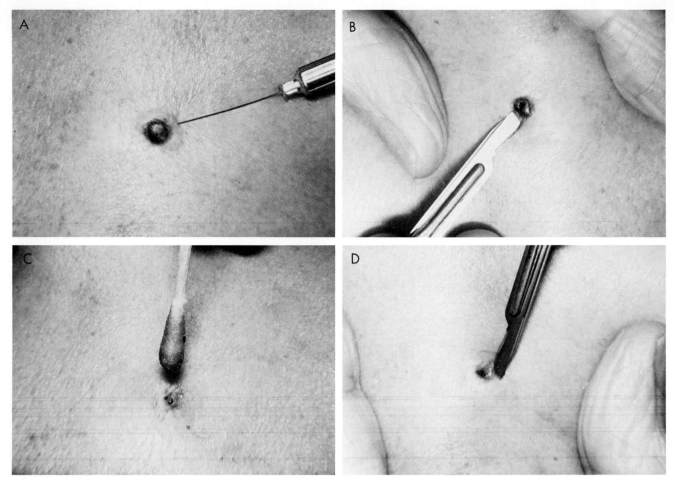

Fig 2–5.—Shave excision of a mole. **A,** injection of local anesthetic. **B,** incision at junction of mole tissue with nor-mal skin. **C,** hemostasis achieved with Monsel's solution. **D,** teasing out the last few deep nevus cells.

Again, hemostasis nearly always is possible to obtain with Monsel's solution or aluminum chloride (Fig 2–5,C). Sometimes, on young children or on people who are having multiple moles removed, pressure alone or the use of Oxycel cotton also are usable hemostatic techniques.

A few cells of mole tissue may be seen deep within the central area after the shave. Many times we elect to leave these cells, knowing that they probably will repigment, but to take them out would involve making a full-thickness dermal wound and would result in a worse scar. If the mole is being removed because it is protuberant and unsightly, we have accomplished our goal with-out creating a bad scar. If the mole is in an area where it is essential that all pigment be removed, we can go back to that area with a curette or, curetting with the #15 scalpel Bard-Parker blade (Fig 2–5,D), try to tease out those last few nevus cells.

With the shave technique, it is advisable to use the scalpel blade to feather the edges of the saucer-like defect created by the shave biopsy. This is a form of minidermabrasion done with the scalpel edge. Hold the skin taut between several fingers and scrape and feather the edges of the defect until the entire area is smooth. This scalpel dermabrasion helps to camouflage the appearance of a dimpled scar. If the mole to be excised is on sebaceous skin, particularly around the nose and central face, it is a good idea to warn the patient that there might be a dimple at the site of the mole removal.

LENTIGINES (LIVER SPOTS)

What the patient may call brown spots, liver spots, moles, etc., usually are one or a combination of several things. A lentigo is a macular (flat), brownish, usually round to oval lesion that appears in multiples over the cheeks (Fig 2–6,A), forehead, and backs of the hands and arms. There probably is a relationship between exposure to sunlight and the development of lentigines.

The histology, as shown in Figure 2–6,B, illustrates that the lesion has a budding of the epidermal rete pegs and increased numbers of melanocytes. It is important to note that this lesion is not exophytic. It is mostly confined to the basal layer of the epidermis. This histology will be contrasted with the histology of the seborrheic keratosis and dermatofibroma—other lesions that have a similar clinical appearance.

For isolated lentigines on the face or the backs of the hands, several techniques of removal are used. Each of these techniques carries a low risk of poor result. One of us (S. J. S.) likes to use the hot cautery, fine-tipped instrument with the setting on very "cool" (Fig 2–6,C). The tip is passed lightly over the lentigo to achieve heat separation of the epidermis from the dermis, much as in the case of a friction blister. The epidermis will literally char and can be wiped off with cotton gauze or with light curetting (Fig 2–6,D). These lesions seldom repigment and almost never scar. Usually, local anesthesia is not necessary, but if the lesion is large (greater than 1.0 cm), local anesthesia is appreciated. If anesthesia is used, it is not necessary to swell the skin below the lesion and push it outward, since only the epidermis is being treated. It is most helpful to have the lesion lying flat. This technique is less successful on the large lesions found on the backs of the hands and arms for reasons we do not completely understand.

The results seem fairly good. It is difficult to tell on lentigines whether there is a recurrence or a new lesion in the same field. There has been little scar formation, if any, in those cases where only the epidermis was removed.

The same technique can be done with light electrodesiccation. The top of the lentigo is gently and lightly desiccated and then the char is wiped off. We find it more difficult to control the depth of the wound with electrodesiccation than with the hot cautery. A sharp ring curette also can be used with a sweeping movement of the curette quickly across the lentigo. For lentigines that have some extension above the surface of the skin, the curette is more likely to be successful. However, it is difficult to sweep the curette quickly and take only the lesion itself with none of the surrounding skin. Chemical escharotics also are successful. Full-strength phenol (88%) and trichloroacetic acid, between 40% and 70%, will eliminate many lentigines and will bleach others. Physicians must differentiate between benign lentigines and precancerous melanomas or premalignant pigmented lesions. If ever in doubt, do a shave or punch biopsy.

Liquid nitrogen spray also is effective in light-complexioned patients. For the best cosmetic results, especially on the hands, terminate the liquid nitrogen

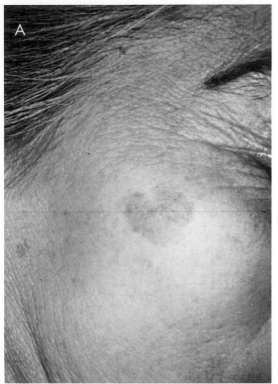

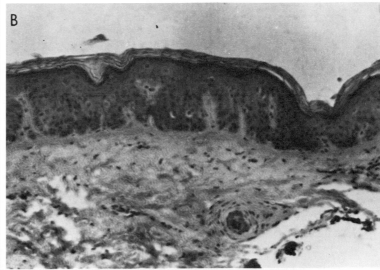

Fig 2–6.—Lentigines. **A,** gross appearance of lesion. **B,** microscopic appearance of lesion. **C,** technique of removal with a fine-tipped cautery instrument. **D,** wiping away the epidermal char with a curette.

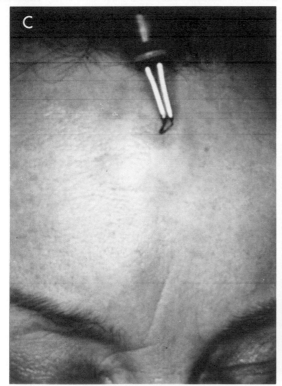

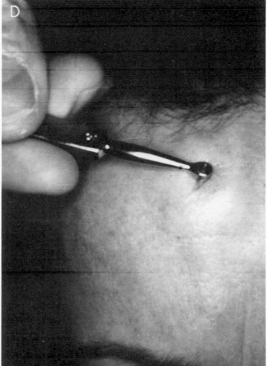

spray as soon as the lesion blanches. Freezing longer than this may cause hypopigmentation rather than simple elimination of the lentigo with a return to normal-colored skin.

Sometimes superficial dermabrasion using a fine diamond fraise or a garnet dental tip without prior freezing anesthesia may be used. On the dorsal hands, these abraded lentigines can be covered with Op-Site dressing to prevent a deeper wound from dehydration.

We are not aware that bleaching creams purchased over the counter or even compounded from a physician's prescription are effective to do any more than occasionally lighten some of these lesions. This is one area where the physician, using a simple surgical technique, offers a result that is quick and has a high rate of success.

SEBORRHEIC KERATOSES

Seborrheic keratosis (Fig 2–7,A) often is an exophytic epidermal lesion, as seen in histologic section (Fig 2–7,B). The size can range from 0.3–0.5-mm to quite large, 1.0–2.0-cm lesions. Sometimes they are warty and darkly pig-

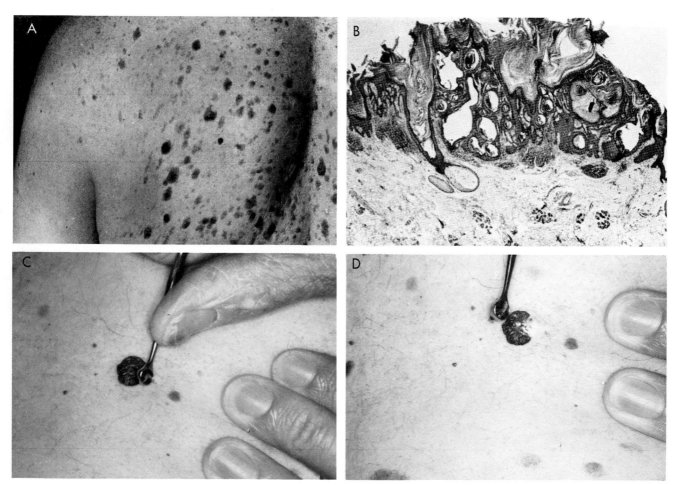

Fig 2–7.—Seborrheic keratosis. **A,** gross appearance. B, microscopic appearance.
C and **D,** removal with appropriately sized curette.

mented and actually are frightening looking. But the experienced eye soon will recognize these lesions and know that only simple superficial techniques are needed for their removal. It would be embarrassing to find that a seborrheic keratosis has been excised and closed primarily with an elaborate technique.

The quickest and easiest way to treat seborrheic keratoses is with an appropriately sized ring curette (Fig 2–7,C), using a sweeping motion through the base of the lesion, as one would use a golf club to hit a ball from a sand trap (Fig 2–7,D). The movement should involve the arm and the wrist, starting behind the lesion and "following through" the other side of the lesion. When this technique is mastered, the keratosis will fly off. Most of the time, if the skin is held taut and if the physician is fast enough, local anesthesia is not needed.

Hemostasis can be obtained with chemical cauterants such as Monsel's solution or aluminum chloride or with Oxycel cotton.

The lack of scarring depends pretty much on the wound depth. If the dermis was not involved, the scar is absent or flat, but some erythema or hypopigmentation may persist.

Whether to obtain histopathology of every seborrheic keratosis is a matter of conjecture. Anyone can be fooled by a melanoma masquerading as a seborrheic keratosis. On the other hand, these lesions are so multiple that histopathology of each one generates excessive cost. We try to approach this problem by sampling two or three of the keratoses of any large group that are removed. We choose the most suspicious-looking lesions to send for histopathology.

Liquid nitrogen freezing, phenol, trichloroacetic acid and electrodesiccation all can be used for removal of seborrheic keratoses. Of these methods, the liquid nitrogen freezing is the most controllable, although not nearly as controllable as the curette or scalpel. The experienced cryotherapist can learn how to raise a blister just below the keratosis, which will allow it to come off at a later date and have minimal problems with scarring. Again, only some dyschromia may result.

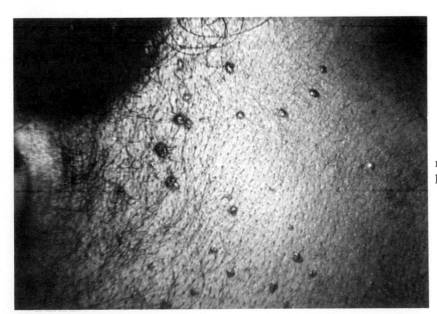

Fig 2–8.—Seborrheic keratoses on the malar prominence of a dark-skinned patient.

Dark-skinned people tend to develop small, black, warty, pedunculated groups of lesions over the malar prominences, lower eyelids, and temple regions (Fig 2–8). These are called dermatosis papulosa nigra and are believed to be a variant of seborrheic keratoses. These can be treated quite quickly and simply with scissor or curet excision and the hemostasis controlled with chemical cauterants. Occasionally, these lesions will heal with a slightly hyperpigmented spot, but the spot is macular and there is little or no real scarring. Another effective method is the use of the hot cautery or the hyfrecator, using the point at the lowest possible current. The distal end of the lesion is touched and allowed to desiccate. Watch it shrivel up until the base is reached and then quickly discontinue the current.

This particular cosmetic problem is so easily treated and so seldom requested. We wonder whether dark-skinned people believe that there is no treatment for them or remember many older members of their family having had these lesions and not having them treated. It is a nice trick to know how to do in case you are asked. This is the kind of problem about which you may gently make the patient aware of the easy treatment available. But do not be surprised if most do not accept your suggestion.

DERMATOFIBROMA

A dermatofibroma is a brownish, firm, dome-shaped lesion that rarely appears on the face (Fig 2–9,A) and upper trunk but usually on the distal extremities, particularly the legs. The histopathology shown in Figure 2–9,B reveals that the lesion is entirely dermal and can extend quite deeply into the dermis.

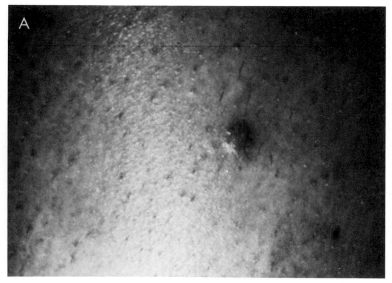

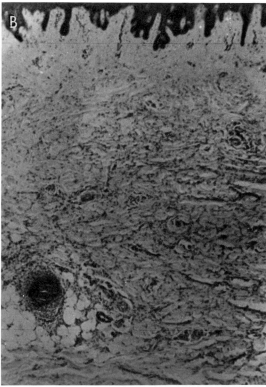

Fig 2–9.—Dermatofibroma. **A,** gross appearance, **B,** microscopic appearance.

It seems to stimulate pigment accumulation in the macrophages above the lesion. There also is an increased deposition of melanin in the overlying epidermis.

We know of only two successful treatments for this lesion. The most successful is liquid nitrogen cryotherapy accomplished with the cryoprobe. It is important to freeze long enough for the ice ball to extend through the full-thickness dermis. After several weeks of healing, an acceptable result ensues, with flattening and softening of the lesion. A small, flat scar, however, will persist. The other treatment is to surgically excise the lesion and to close primarily. This involves trading a flat, not too obvious lesion for a surgical scar. Most of the time, these lesions are not treated, and the patients will accept your reassurance that they are benign. Excision usually leaves a blemish more unsightly than the dermatofibroma itself.

SEBACEOUS HYPERPLASIA

Sebaceous hyperplasia (Fig 2–10,A) is common in middle-aged and older patients. It presents as shiny, yellowish, irregularly shaped, elevated papules,

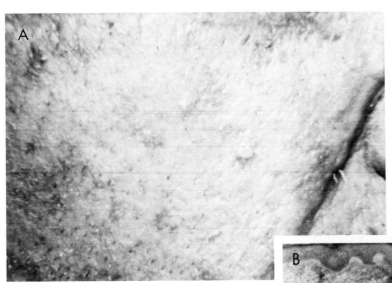

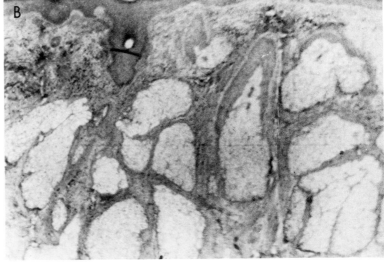

Fig 2–10.—Sebaceous hyperplasia. **A,** gross appearance. **B,** microscopic appearance.

usually on the face. Once the physician learns to recognize the creamy color with some red tinges, the differential diagnosis is not difficult. Figure 2–10,B shows the histology of sebaceous hyperplasia. It is entirely a dermal lesion, possibly with some thinning of the epidermis if the lesion is protuberant. Consequently, a shave type of excision is not successful, and excision with primary closure would present problems with scarring. We believe that the treatment of choice is full-strength phenol (88%) applied with a Q-tip or wooden stick exactly to the area of sebaceous hyperplasia. If an open phenol peeling is unsuccessful, a repeated peeling can be done one to three months later, using tape occlusion for 24–48 hours to increase the depth of the wound. Trichloroacetic acid, 40%–60%, also can be used, but the penetration of the wound is not as deep. Equally effective is touching each lesion with the cautery or epilating current as described for milia.

The risks and side effects of phenol peeling usually are not a problem because such small amounts are used on such small areas of the body. However, the patient needs to be reminded of the possibility that the area can be hyperpigmented or hypopigmented and that there will be persistent erythema for three to six weeks. We also remind the patients that we know that we are making a chemical wound but we cannot guarantee the results, since we have no real control over the depth of the penetration of the phenol wound.

Sometimes there are large areas of sebaceous hyperplasia rather than discrete lesions. If the lesions are quite large, some of the risks and side effects of a larger area of phenol peeling must be considered. Consult the chapter 3 on chemical peels for discussion of the risks and side effects of large-area peels.

XANTHELASMA (XANTHOMAS)

Xanthelasma is another common benign lesion that can become extremely unsightly. The yellow plaques around the upper and lower eyelids, but particularly the medial upper eyelids (Fig 2–11,A), are the most commonly seen and the most cosmetically distracting. We believe that the treatment of choice for xanthelasmas on the eyelids is excision and primary closure. Fortunately, there often is redundant skin in the eyelid, so that the area heals with minimal exposure of the scar, provided that proper surgical technique is used.

In cases where excision is not reasonable or when xanthelasma recurs after excision, trichloroacetic acid, 50%–100%, is quite effective. The xanthelasma is painted with trichloroacetic acid, using a pointed wooden applicator stick to which a small amount of cotton has been tightly wrapped (see Fig 2–11,A). The applicator is dipped into the trichloroacetic acid and then wrung out by rolling pressure on the inside of the neck of the bottle. This dripless applicator then is used to apply trichloroacetic acid carefully to only the xanthomas. Sufficient trichloroacetic acid is applied so that the whole lesion shows an even, white-frosting appearance (Fig 2–11,B). A cotton gauze pad, soaked in cool tap water, then is applied to dilute residual surface trichloroacetic acid (Fig 2–11,C). Crusts (Fig 2–11,D) are off within two weeks. A flat, pink scar usually forms but usually is not seen unless the eyelid tissue is spread and the scar sought (Fig 2–11,E). Retreatment is often necessary for complete removal.

Xanthomas elsewhere on the body seldom are a cosmetic problem but more one of function. Surgical excision with primary closure still is the treatment of choice, but other problems such as protecting the function of joints and invasion into important underlying anatomical structures need to be considered; however, they are beyond the scope of this text.

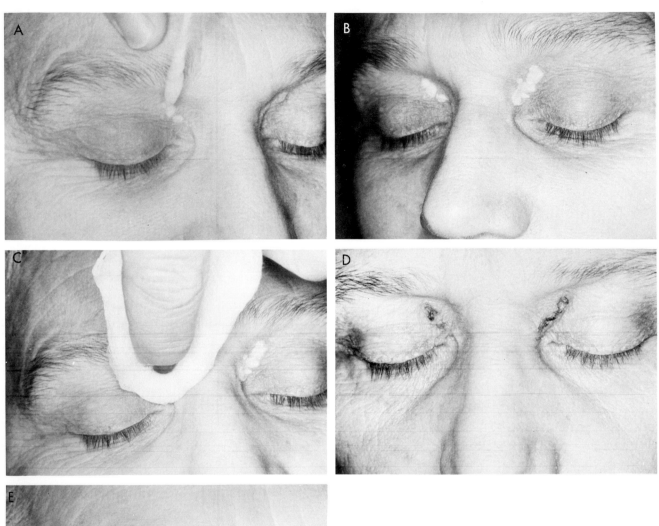

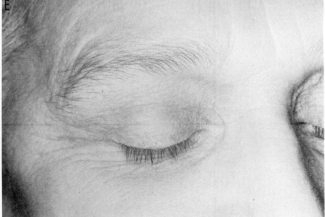

Fig 2–11.—Xanthomas. **A,** lesion on medial upper eyelid is painted with trichloroacetic acid. **B,** entire lesion with an even, white-frosting appearance. **C,** cotton gauze pad soaked in water applied. **D,** appearance of crusts, which slough off within two weeks. **E,** appearance following crust slough.

CHLOASMA (MELASMA)

This unfortunate pigmentary problem (Fig 2–12), found mostly in women of childbearing age and occasionally in men, can be a serious cosmetic problem. Our treatments are poor at best. We generally try one of several bleaching preparations in addition to the use of good sunscreens to decrease the intensity of the pigmentation. Over the years, the most popular bleaching agents in the dermatologic literature have included 3%–6% hydroquinone in various creams and ointment bases, 6% hydroquinone in conjunction with a topical corticosteroid and retinoic acid, and the use of 3%–6% hydroquinone mixed in Neutrogena-N vehicle. Many patients have been helped by these preparations. However, the results usually are slow and partial, and many other patients are quite unhappy with the results.

Some physicians have found that application of 25%–35% trichloroacetic acid at two- to four-week intervals peels off some of the pigmented stratum corneum. We estimate that a maximum of 25% additional improvement probably could be obtained through this technique.

Chloasma has also been treated successfully by dermabrasion or phenol tape peels. It is absolutely essential for both the physician and patient to realize that all of these treatments for melasma carry the risk that the patient will come out looking worse. We all know of examples in which peels, dermabrasions, and bleaching agents have caused increased hyperpigmentation. This unfortunate circumstance becomes more unfortunate if the patient was not very carefully advised of the risk. The risk and the physician's cautions must be documented on the chart. This is one of the examples in which we list the risks on the chart and ask the patients to sign our notation on the chart indicating that they have read it and understand what is noted.

The discussion in this book on the use of cosmetics is especially helpful when one is confronted with patients with chloasma. We strongly urge all physicians who encounter patients with cosmetic problems to read carefully the discussions about cosmetics, since your work with the patients is greatly

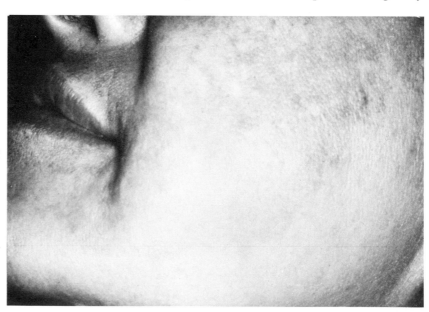

Fig 2–12.—Chloasma in female of childbearing age.

improved if you are able to give specific answers on how best to disguise their problems.

LIPOMAS

Lipomas that protrude and are obvious are unsightly. To the lay person, they can appear malignant or can indicate some sort of disease process in ad-

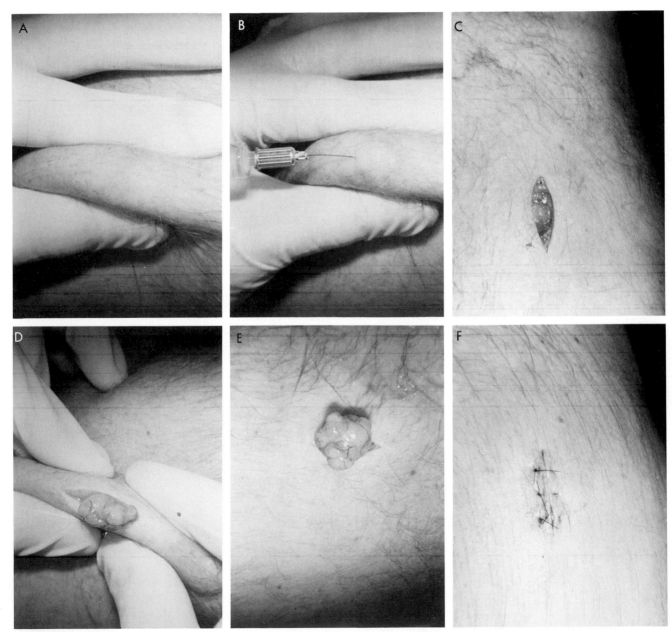

Fig 2–13.—Lipoma. Technique of excision. **A,** grasp the lipoma between the thumb and forefinger. **B,** anesthetize the skin overlaying the tumor. **C,** incise through full-thickness of skin to level of lipoma. **D,** pressure by thumb and forefinger on bulk of lipoma causes it to extrude, often like a mass of grapes **(E). F,** suture of incision.

dition to being unsightly. They are particularly noticeable on the upper trunk, shoulders, anterior chest, and arms of women and on the lower arms of men. Sometimes they occur on the face.

The best treatment for a lipoma is to excise it. The best technique is to grasp the lipoma between the thumb and forefinger in one hand (Fig 2–13,A), anesthetize the skin overlying the lipoma using the other hand (Fig 2–13,B), and not release the grip on the tumor. The scalpel incision is made through the full-thickness skin to the level of the lipoma (Fig 2–13,C), but only one-fourth to one-half the length of the lipoma. As the skin opens up, gentle but firm, steady pressure is exerted on the bulk of the lipoma with the thumb and forefinger (Fig 2–13,D). Often the lipoma will extrude like a mass of grapes or a piece of liver through the incision (Fig 2–13,E). The remaining surgical problems are simply ones of hemostasis and obliteration of dead space or further excision of atrophic skin overlying the lipoma (Fig 2–13,F).

At other times, the lipoma will not extrude on its own and will need to be dissected out. Sometimes gentle, blunt scissor dissection separating the lipoma from the overlying skin will be enough that the thumb and forefinger pressure then can extrude the tumor.

Some lipomas are too large (4.0–5.0 cm) for this type of technique, or the skin over them is too thick or taut, such as on the thigh or midback. In these cases, after the primary incision is made, the lipoma is simply dissected out, much as for an epidermal cyst. It is important to remember that the large dead space that is created by the lipoma can be a problem because of late bleeding or seroma formation. Also, if the skin overlying the lipoma is atrophic, the side-to-side healing through the incision line may result in a poor or depressed, widened scar. With atrophic skin, it is best to excise the skin back to normal skin and then bury sutures, as necessary, to obliterate the dead space before the primary skin repair is made. Liposuction is an excellent new technique for large (>4 cm diameter) lipomas.

The patients should be advised that with lipoma surgery they are exchanging an unsightly lump for a surgical scar. If the lipoma is in the anterior chest or the shoulders of a female, she needs to be warned that sometimes normal healing in this area results in a hypertrophic scar. Most of the time, the exchange of the protruding lipoma for a surgical scar is beneficial.

SYRINGOMA

Syringomas (Fig 2–14,A) are hamartomatous lesions differentiating toward sweat ducts. The histology of syringoma is shown in Figure 2–14,B. Obviously, from the histology, the involvement is within the dermis and the lesion itself can extend anywhere from the subcutaneous fat to immediately below the epidermis.

The only treatment we know for these lesions is surgical excision. Usually they are multiple and are mostly on the lower eyelids. Consequently, surgery seldom is indicated because multiple small incisions would have to be made and closed primarily or large sections of lower-eyelid tissue would need to be removed. This is not, however, an area amenable to loss of eyelid tissue. If a particular lesion is infected, irritated, or annoying, the trade-off for surgical excision might become worthwhile. But this is an isolated case. Most of the time, patients are not encouraged to have treatment.

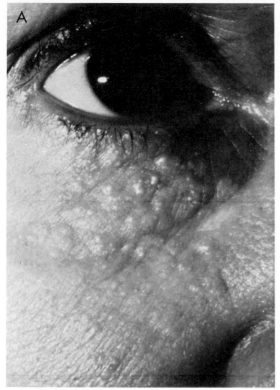

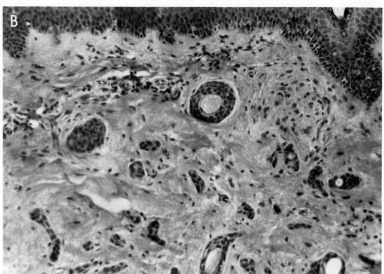

Fig 2–14.—Syringoma.
A, gross appearance.
B, microscopic appearance.

CHERRY ANGIOMA

These lesions usually are 0.2–0.5 cm in diameter and are made up of mature ectatic vessels. They are found mostly on the upper trunk, upper extremities, and occasionally on the face and other areas. Many times they resolve spontaneously; at other times, they seem to persist and occasionally grow. Most adults are satisfied with the answer that the lesions are benign lesions that occasionally will resolve and have no potential for malignancy. Others may request treatment if the lesions are isolated and on a fairly young patient in an exposed area.

Treatment is by shave excision with local anesthesia. Light desiccation of the base occasionally is necessary, since there often is an active vessel that is hard to stop with chemical cauterants. Only occasionally is there a small scar left at the site. Electrodesiccation and cryotherapy can be used successfully, particularly for multiple lesions. All three of these methods, used carefully, can provide excellent results.

UNWANTED HAIR

The mustache area, the chin and cheeks, the sideburn area, and the area around the breasts are those from which women most want hair removed. Occasionally, men will request removal of hair when they become frustrated with chronic pseudofolliculitis or irritation from shaving. Also, some men may want to have removed those few remaining miniaturizing hairs on their forehead, which give evidence of the former location of their frontal hairline.

There are four treatment choices for unwanted hair: bleaching, shaving, depilation, and epilation. Bleaching can be done with any of the standard bleaching agents and merely removes the dark color of the hair. Shaving or clipping is good if the hairs are fairly isolated and are not too numerous. The problem that arises when shaving a large number of hairs that are close together, particularly on the face, is that a stubble is created. There is no increase in pigmentation, size, or speed of regrowth after shaving. Many patients resist shaving because the stubble is more noticeable, more difficult to cover with makeup, and has a rough feeling whereas these same hairs with a two- or three-month growth are soft, somewhat bleached, tapered, and lie flat.

Depilation can be done with a number of over-the-counter products sold that generally contain thioglycolates. Application of these chemicals to the hair weakens the hair shaft at the surface of the skin and it then can be wiped off at that level.

Epilation can be performed in several ways. Tweezing or plucking causes no permanent problems and is an acceptable way to remove small numbers of isolated, large hairs. Occasionally, tweezing and plucking causes a complete hair follicle to come out and not regrow.

Another epilatory method uses heated wax, which is applied to the skin and allowed to harden. After it has hardened, the entire sheet is pulled off and, thus, all of the hairs are pulled out. This gives one of the best cosmetic appearances and has the longest-lasting effect, since the telogen hairs and anagen hairs are both removed at the same time. It also usually pulls the hairs out somewhat below the surface of the skin and, thus, the effect will last longer. Hairs have to be a certain length to be effective for wax epilation. Therefore, it cannot be used on extremely short hairs. This is just the time when the stubble appearance is difficult to cover with makeup. Many patients are not eager to apply the wax epilators, since it is something of a nuisance involving adjusting the temperature to be hot enough to work without irritating the skin. These patients have the process done at a beauty parlor. There definitely are patients whose facial skin is far too easily irritated to use wax epilation.

An electrologist can provide permanent epilation. Occasionally we will epilate the large hairs in an intradermal nevus or one or two large hairs that are particularly disturbing to the patient. However, the procedure is time-consuming and probably not the best use of office time. We recommend that the physician make contact with a good electrologist in his area to whom he can refer his patients. There seems to be no shortcut to finding a reputable and talented practitioner in your area. The best thing seems to be to refer your patients and then to follow-up their results carefully.

Permanent epilation is time-consuming, often taking up to two years, and can become expensive, but it is permanent a certain amount of the time, and with repeated visits can offer good improvement for selected patients.

If the pain of epilation is a great problem for patients, we suggest that they first come to our office, have the area anesthetized, and then go immediately to the electrologist for therapy. We also believe that it is an acceptable and valuable service to patients to have an electrologist work part time in your office or in the same office building. That way, the patients can avail themselves of your referral immediately, local anesthesia can be easily facilitated, and you can carefully follow up the work of the electrologist.

3 / Chemical Peels

HISTORY

Peeling, as we in the United States know it, probably came to us from Europe, where Gypsies passed the formulas down from one to another. It was from the immigration of German dermatologists who came to the United States in the 1920s and 1930s that we trace our exposure to the technique. The work of Dr. Thomas Baker of Miami elevated present-day face peeling to a generally accepted medical procedure.[1-6] His classic studies on the various combinations of formulas for face peeling, the safety studies for hepatotoxicity and nephrotoxicity, and his careful long-term follow-up of hundreds of patients established this procedure as a scientific one that could be offered with favorable risk-to-benefit ratio for the patient. The formula for creating a phenol mixture on which Baker eventually settled has become one of the most popular formulas in use today.

Peeling, with both physical and chemical modalities, has long been an important method in the treatment of acne. Twenty-percent trichloroacetic acid (TCA), β-naphthol, various enzymes, resorcinol 20%, and salicylic acid all have been used to remove the stratum corneum around impacted follicles. The effect is helpful but temporary, and is used less today than in the past.

Light also has been used to produce a similar desquamation. Cold quartz machines, which produce 95% of the light rays in the 250-nm range, and the sunburn spectrum of the ultraviolet range have been used frequently both in and out of the office to produce a superficial desquamation over the acne-involved skin. These methods are clearly salutary but now are used less frequently.

DYNAMICS

Little is known about the true cause-and-effect relationship between what the peeling agent does and the effect of its use. Many studies have been performed on the safety of these agents, as discussed below. But the investigation as to how chemical wounds improve the appearance of the skin has not gone past the study of these wounds. Some work has been done on animals, and most of the work done on humans is spotty, since it is difficult to obtain multiple biopsy specimens from the sun-exposed areas (the face) of patients who are seeking an improved cosmetic appearance.

In a study performed by one of us (S. J. S.), the skin of the lateral and posterior surface of the neck of a 55-year-old man was used for serial biopsies of the early and the late postpeeling changes.[7] In that study, the effects of occlusion and nonocclusion on both thin, slightly sun-damaged, and thick, severely sun-damaged skin were compared. The results indicated that the depth of the wound was related to the strength of the agent used. Baker's formula

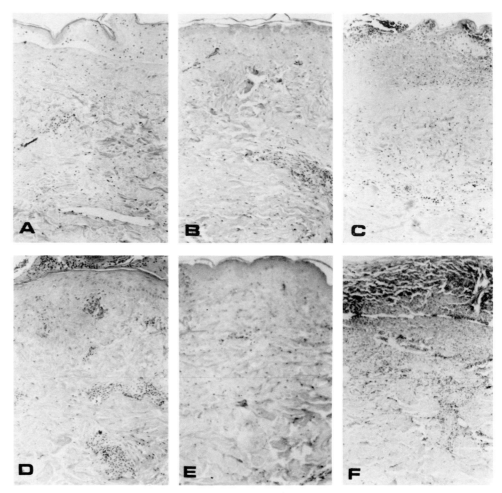

Fig 3–1.—Nonsundamaged skin, three days after treatment with trichloroacetic acid, **A** and **D;** 100% phenol, **B** and **E;** Baker's formula phenol mixture, **C** and **F.** Sections **A, B,** and **C** were left open; sections **D, E,** and **F** were occluded 24 hours.

phenol mixture wounded deeper than full-strength (88%) phenol, which wounded deeper than 50% trichloroacetic acid. The effect of tape occlusion was to increase the depth of the wound for all three agents (Fig 3–1). The sundamaged skin with the thickened elastotic band in the upper dermis wounded in a manner similar to that of non–sun-damaged skin, except that the elastotic band did not seem to offer any barrier to the effect of the chemical agents, and the overall thickness of the wound produced was deeper than that of the non–sun-damaged skin (Fig 3–2).

The thickness of the eschar that developed during healing and the overall time needed for complete healing also were proportional to the depth of the wound produced. How these various depths of wounds apply clinically to the selection of which agent to use and for which indication will be discussed below. The histologic studies did reveal, however, that the healed skin 120 days after wounding with these three peeling agents is different from nonpeeled skin in two aspects: the thickness of the regenerated papillary dermis is related

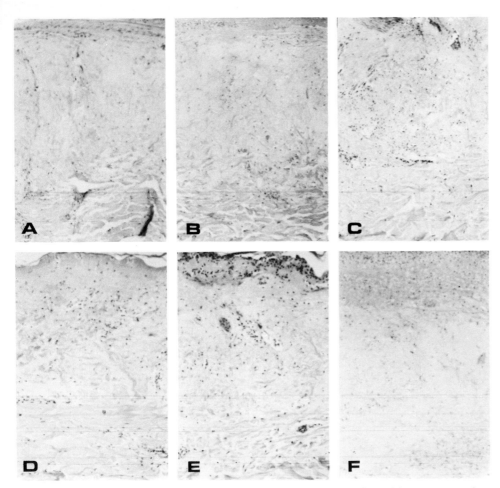

Fig 3–2.—Sundamaged skin, three days after treatment with trichloroacetic acid, **A** and **D**; 100% phenol, **B** and **E**; Baker's formula phenol mixture, **C** and **F**. Sections **A**, **B**, and **C** were left open; sections **D**, **E**, and **F** were occluded 24 hours.

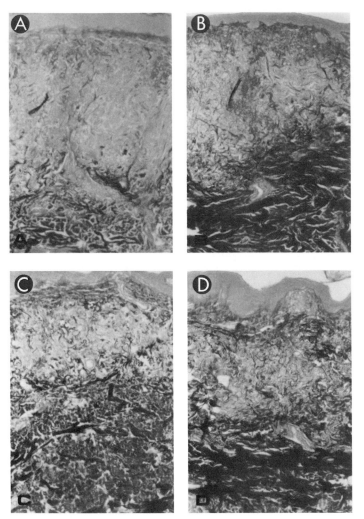

Fig 3–3.—Colloidal iron stains on sundamaged skin; section **A,** a normal control; sections **B, C,** and **D,** 120 days after treatment with trichloroacetic acid, 100% phenol, and Baker's formula phenol mixture, respectively, and occluded for 24 hours.

to the strength of the wounding agent used; and the stronger agents produce a thicker, new papillary dermis (Fig 3–3). For the deeper wounds, the regenerated papillary dermis was thicker than before the use of the wounding agent. The second change is that a middle to upper dermal "scar" develops. This band of dermis, which stains heavily with elastic stains, is histologically different, replaces the elastotic band in sun-damaged skin, and develops *de novo* in non–sun-damaged skin (Fig 3–4). The thickness of this band and the amount of elastic stain that it picks up is also proportional to the strength of the wounding agent used. What effects the thickened papillary dermis and the "dermal scar" have on the cosmetic appearance of the postpeeled skin is not known.

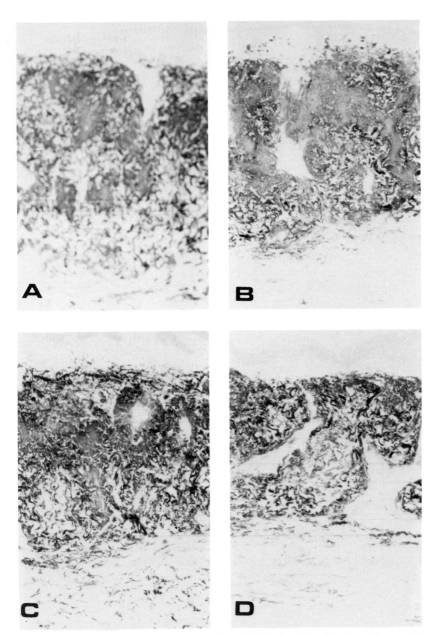

Fig 3–4.—Nonsundamaged skin, stained with Verhoeff's elastic stain; section **A,** a normal control; section **B,** 60 days after treatment with 100% phenol left open; section **C,** 60 days after treatment with 100% phenol occluded for 24 hours; section **D,** 60 days after treatment with Baker's formula phenol mixture occluded for 24 hours.

TOXICITY

There are good studies on animals and man to prove that phenolic compounds are quickly absorbed percutaneously.[8, 9] In animals, the absorbed phenol rapidly produced generalized stimulation of motor nerve endings or spinal motor centers with possible central depression. There also is hemoglobinuria, possibly owing to widespread intravascular hemolysis. The severity of these effects was markedly influenced by the dilution of phenol with water.

The highest concentrations of phenol did not necessarily produce the most serious toxicity. A combination of phenol and water 2:1 was the most toxic. This same type of phenol concentration effect has also been shown clinically in human beings[10] by the observation that a mixture that has a final concentration of phenol of 50%–60% produces the deepest wound when compared with full-strength (88%) phenol.

It has been demonstrated that application of phenol to the face may result in an immediate arrhythmia. This may relate to the "face splash reflex." A crude, effective means of slowing down the heart rate with some arrhythmias is to take the patient's face and splash it into a pan of cold water. Although crude, it often is successful, since there is a natural reflex to slow the heart rate. This reflex exists in animals, too; e.g., in the duck. When its face is thrust into the water, the heart rate slows down, supposedly to prepare the duck for a long period of swimming underwater.

Cardiac toxicity has also been shown by clinical studies. Truppman, et al., have demonstrated that rapidly applied phenolic mixtures will lead to life-threatening cardiac arrhythmias.[14] These arrhythmias did not seem to be related to the age of the patient; the amount of anesthesia and, thus, perceived pain; or to the clinical reasons for the application of the peel. They seemed to be related only to the speed with which the phenol was applied.

A damaged epidermis theoretically allows a much more rapid penetration of the phenol than nondamaged skin, and it is assumed that some phenol is trapped within the necrotic bands of the various layers of the skin. Evidence is lacking to prove that the skin damaged by phenol acts as its own barrier or as a trap for slow release of more of the cauterant.

Patients who have survived industrial or accidental cutaneous exposures of phenol to large areas have developed nephrotoxicity and hepatotoxicity. These problems have not resulted from the small, controlled doses of phenol used in a medical situation.

Industrial decontamination studies with phenol and phenolic compounds have not been discussed widely in the medical literature, but they might be helpful for the physician who inadvertently applies more phenol than he had planned or if there is an accidental spilling or exposure of this compound to the patient, the office staff, or the physician himself. Recent studies indicate that the best decontamination procedure is to flood the area exposed to the phenol with propylene gylcol or with glycerol.[8, 9, 11]These areas should be swabbed and rubbed liberally with cotton swabs soaked in the glycerol or propylene glycol. In the case of accidental spill or excess application of phenol, the patient should be taken to the appropriate medical facility, where cardiac monitoring can be performed and support can be administered in case of cardiac arrhythmias, shock, or convulsions.

Another agent used is polyethylene glycol 300 or 400. Polyethylene glycol is viscous at normal ambient temperatures, but may solidify in cold weather. A mixture of polyethylene glycol with industrial methylated spirit is available in a 2:1 volume mixture and can be stored at room temperature for long periods. There also is evidence that olive oil may somewhat stop the penetration, skin injury, and systemic toxic reaction to phenol, but its oiliness and slipperiness make it quite difficult to use in a hospital or office. Although it has not been standard medical practice to have polyethylene glycol in industrial methylated spirit at hand, the literature for industrial safety and accident prevention supports this as the only true mixture that will decrease systemic intoxication and decrease the localized injury to the skin.

INDICATIONS AND TECHNIQUE

There are several different chemicals or chemical mixtures that we use commonly for face peeling. There also are several different indications. The indications for and the technique of the Baker's formula phenol peel will be described in full detail. Afterward, the indications for and the variations in technique will be described for the other materials used.

The indication for the Baker's phenol peel[12] occluded is almost limited to sun-damaged skin. This technique is predictably reliable for improving the appearance of the fine cross-hatched wrinkling, crepey appearance, and irregular pigmentation of the skin on the face. Surprisingly, some of the creases (those folds secondary to muscle pull from the movement of the mouth, cheek, or eyelids or from gravity's pull) also will be partially or completely removed with this technique. Obviously, the creases return, but sometimes their improved appearance will last for several years. The elastotic changes in the skin are completely "corrected" if they are shallow and they are nearly completely erased if they are deep. The lasting effect of peeling has been shown in biopsy studies of patients who had peels followed by face-lifts as long as 13 years later; the peeled skin retains that "dermal scar" and the improved clinical appearance, provided that the patient did not have further sun damage.[13]

The effects of the peel on pigmentary lesions, such as melasma and intradermal nevi, is unpredictable. But with the recent knowledge that melasma may have different depths of pigment dispersement, certain cases may predictably respond to treatment by peeling. Often the nevi and melasma will be lightened. However, equally often the surrounding skin will become more hypopigmented, so that the pigmentary lesions will be contrasted more and thus will be more obvious. To use the phenol face peel for any indication other than sun damage invites unpredictable results.

The technique for the Baker's formula phenol peel is quite similar to that used for full-strength phenol or any of the trichloroacetic acid peels. After the patient has been properly informed of the procedure, prognosis, and risks, both in previous consultations and before the administration of any preoperative medications, he or she is brought to the office surgery room. Preoperative photos are taken and any further questions the patient may have are answered. Postoperative care is discussed with the patient, and matters such as how the patient will be taken home, who will care for the patient during the first 24 hours, etc., will be discussed. We ask the patient not to wear makeup on the day of surgery and also to cleanse the face well with soap and water the night before surgery and the morning of surgery. Most of the time this is adequate preoperative preparation for a face peel. If there is any hint of oiliness or residual makeup, we will again wash the face in the office. If, however, the face is completely dry and free from oil, there is no reason one cannot proceed. Some physicians believe that the face should be degreased and use ether or acetone. There are beliefs (unproved) that the oil on the face will hinder the penetration of the escharotic agent, which results in unequal peel. Others believe that if the peel is to be occluded with tape, the degreasing of the face insures even adherence of the tape. We certainly agree that a degreased face will allow the tape to stick more easily, but sticking of the tape never has been a problem for us. A good soap and water cleansing is quite adequate.

Preoperative analgesia varies with the individual physician's preference, the depth of the peel to be applied, and the patient's own anxieties and preferences. Many patients who are well motivated can be given no more than 75–150 mg of meperidine hydrochloride (Demerol) IM and 10 mg of diazepam (Valium) sublingually and do quite well throughout the entire procedure. Others require Valium orally and sublingually and occasionally intravenously (IV). Various combinations of diazepam, meperidine, and fentanyl citrate administered in small doses IV produce rapid sedation of such a depth that the patient stays in a state of sleep but can easily be aroused by voice command.

If a cardiac monitor is available, it is wise to use it for any phenol face peel because of the risks of cardiac arrhythmias. If available, an IV line with 5% dextrose in water (D5W) can be placed. This gives the physician easy access for further administration of analgesic drugs as well as a quick intravascular entrance in case of complications. If arrhythmias develop, stop any further application of the phenol until the cardiac rate has been regular for 15 minutes. Then apply the phenol mixture in smaller increments, timed further apart. Lidocaine (Xylocaine) can be injected IV in 5–10-mg doses to control arrhythmias.

Field block anesthesia for the entire face can be achieved with the longer acting agents such as bupivacaine (Marcaine) or etidocaine (Duranest). The field block, if successful, gives the patient a great deal of relief during the surgery and for several hours afterward. The pain from the face peel seems to last only four to six hours and then stops abruptly. This is an almost universal event, and patients can be told with assurance that the postoperative pain will cease that evening. Since pain at nighttime is less well tolerated than pain in the daylight hours, we try to do face peels in the morning and advise the patient that before bedtime the pain will be gone. We have had patients who had the face field anesthesia and told us that they had no pain until the next day, when they experienced the usual discomfort from swelling, oozing, and crusting.

The Baker phenol mixture is a combination of an epidermolytic (in this case, croton oil), a soap (in this case, Septisol) that is used as a surfactant, and phenol, with the mixture formulated so that the final concentration of phenol is in the 50%–55% range (Table 3–1). The mixture is not miscible and separates in the container. Consequently, the material needs to be stirred well with the

TABLE 3–1.—BAKER'S PHENOL
MIXTURE

3 ml U.S.P. phenol
2 ml tap water
9 gtt liquid soap (Septisol)
3 gtt croton oil

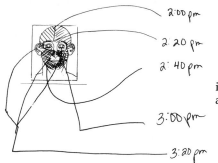

Fig 3–5.—Face peel chart indicating times at which various areas were treated.

cotton applicators before each application to the patient. Although it is not necessary, we always make up the mixture fresh and individually for each surgery.

Cotton-tipped applicators, not rayon-tipped applicators, are the routine in our office. However, other physicians have used variations by adapting web roll cotton to the ends of wooden dowels or the wooden end of small paint-brushes. Sometimes the larger cotton-tipped swabs used in proctology have been utilized. However, in the light of recent evidence that the rapid application of the phenol is the factor that is cardiotoxic, we feel safer applying it slowly and comfortably with the use of ordinary cotton-tipped applicators.[14] For narrow areas of the face, such as around the alar fold or on the eyelids, we will use one applicator (Plate I–A). For broad planes and fields on the facial skin, we will place two to three applicators abreast and paint over the entire area with sweeping, broad strokes of the applicators side by side (Plate I–B).

It is important to do only one cosmetic area at a time, and the boundaries of the units may vary if the face is extremely wrinkled or there is a redundancy of the skin with creases and folds. One can start on the forehead on one side and then the other, then move to the lateral cheek, the medial cheek, the chin, etc.; or one can start on the chin and work up one side entirely and then do the other. It is not critical, except that an hour to an hour and a half be allowed for an entire face peel with any phenol mixture. We try to do one area and leave the patient with the assistant so that we are not tempted to hurry. On the chart, a notation is made of the time each section is done. For example, the chart will say, "10:15, right chin," and the next entry will say, "10:30, left chin," etc. (Fig 3–5).

If the skin of the face is severely wrinkled and redundant, the amount of surface area is greater. In the areas of these wrinkles, an entire cosmetic unit should not be peeled at one application; rather, the cosmetic unit should be divided into several smaller ones with the wrinkles stretched out. Sometimes a single cotton applicator is needed to work deeply into each crease and wrinkle so that the frost is even over the entire face at one time or another.

For the application of the escharotic, we dip the cotton-tipped applicators into the mixture and stir well. Then the cotton tips are pressed dry against the side of the dish (Plate I–C), aligned abreast, and rubbed over the patient's skin with smooth, regular strokes. When the Baker's formula is used, frosting takes place within a few seconds (Plate I–D). The entire cosmetic unit can be peeled and an even frost obtained by going over the area again until the even, deep white frost is evident. Another safety technique is to limit the amount of phenol to only that contained in three cotton-tipped applicators. For example, we will use the three cotton-tipped applicators abreast with one dip into the phenol mixture and be able to frost one-half of the chin, one-half of the cheek, one-half of the forehead, etc. This then becomes the total amount we will apply in that 10- to 15-minute period. The application is continued until the entire face is done.

The agent must be taken beyond the vermilion border (Plate I–E). Peeling up to the vermilion border does not wound lip wrinkles deeply enough and may leave an untreated line around the lip that is quite unsightly. There is no reason why the lips themselves cannot be peeled. Many of the rhitides of the perioral region extend right onto the lip, and these will respond to the peeling agents the same as the rest of the skin. It is in these radiating creases that the lipstick runs, creating the telltale red streaks of the upper lip area. These creases must be treated fully for good results. We peel right up to the oral commissure. The same is true around hair-bearing areas: we peel into the hairline (Plate I–F), sideburns, and eyebrows (Plate I–G). Hair is not lost, and even if it were, it probably would be just a telogen effluvium and would regrow. It is important to peel the tragus and the ear lobe. Both of these often are wrinkled the same as the face, and failure to treat them draws attention to them.

Because they hurt so much, we always do the eyelids last. There are different opinions as to how strong an agent should be used on the eyelids because of the thin skin, which easily can develop a full-thickness wound. Some physicians will use only a 20% or 30% trichloroacetic acid on the eyelids. We routinely use full-strength (88%) phenol non-occluded for both the upper and lower eyelids. We rarely will use the Baker's formula for the eyelids, although other physicians do so quite successfully. We have seen full-thickness slough of eyelid tissue with the Baker's formula peel (in each case, these healed without noticeable scarring or permanent morbidity). However, the results of a full-strength (88%) phenol open peel are adequate, and even the results with a 20% or 30% trichloroacetic acid peel usually are an improvement.

The technique for the eyelids is to stand at the head of the table and lean over the patient so that the physician and patient are face to face. Ask the patient to follow your eyes. A single cotton-tipped applicator is dipped into full-strength phenol and wrung out dry. Apply it to the lower eyelid with the patient's eyes open and following your eyes. We tell patients that they can blink all they want, but then they open their eyes to stare again directly at our eyes. An assistant stands ready to blot any tears. It takes just a few seconds to peel the entire lower lid to up to 1 mm of the ciliary margin. This is followed by application to the other lower eyelid and then the upper eyelids. We allow about five to ten minutes between each eyelid.

The use of eye drops or ointments to protect the eyes is unnecessary. The biggest problem with doing eyelids is that the patient will tear. The escharotic agent will be diluted by the tears, become ineffective, and thus leave a spot or streak of ineffectively peeled skin. If by accident some of the escharotic agent should get into the eye, it is immediately diluted by the tears and further diluted by flooding with water. We have found that we have the best control simply by obtaining the patient's cooperation and using only one "dry" cotton-tipped applicator at a time. This area of the face is the most sensitive to the peeling, and the patient who has tolerated the rest of the procedure may find this part almost intolerable.

There is a lot of discussion about "neutralizing" the escharotic agent with either water or alcohol. There is no true chemical reaction that takes place with alcohol and trichloroacetic acid or phenol, merely a phenomenon of dilution. The burning that the patient feels at the application of the phenol is transient— it usually is gone within 10 to 15 seconds. We ordinarily apply a cool compress over the peeled area mostly because it feels cooling to the patient and gives the patient the reassurance of receiving constant attention (Plate I–H). We suspect that it has no effect either way on the results of the peel.

When peeling along the lateral canthal region and the temple, consider that in some patients the closed upper eyelid forms a small channel leading right to the lateral canthus. Sometimes the escharotic agent can be picked up in this channel and pulled by capillary attraction into the eye. We carefully hold the eye open when we are peeling around the lateral canthus and then follow with the application of water. This insures that the capillary action does not pull the agent into the eye.

Sometimes blending the depth of the peel from the face to the neck is difficult. With the patient lying down, the effects of gravity are not always perceived. The skin along the jaw shifts up and down depending upon how much jowl there is. The peel should be carried below the jaw on to the submandibular or neck skin so that the transition line between the peeled and unpeeled skin will be hidden. Therefore, we like to do peels with patients in a semisitting position to allow for the effects of gravity. We can go back, however, and redo the jawline in order to bring the pigment changes into the shadow of the jaw, but it often is not as even as when done at the initial peeling.

As with all peels strong enough to sufficiently affect wrinkling, treatment of the neck is most difficult because you do not know where to stop. A woman will draw a line at the bottom of her neck in a semi-circular fashion. This is fine if she always will wear a round collar, but you can be sure that she has some V-necked clothing. If you do the V of her neck, she will look different when she wears a dress with a wider opening or a bathing suit. Althogh peeling of various parts of the body can be done, in our experience it is best to limit it to the face and occasionally the upper neck because of the ability to hide the difference naturally in skin below the jawline. Palpate the jaw or have the patient in the sitting position to note the effect of gravity. Bring the peel down to below the jawline so that if a line of difference exists between the color of the face and the neck, it will be hidden in the shadow of the jaw.

Approximately 20 to 40 minutes after the face has been peeled, it begins to hurt severely. Some people describe this as burning, others describe it as severe heat, and others simply say that it hurts. Thus, most of the time throughout the peel, the patients are not in a great deal of pain, but toward the end of the procedure they become uncomfortable. At that time more analgesia can be added, either IV or IM, or the patient can be given codeine orally.

In many patients the skin inferior to the lateral eyebrow is not thin eyelid skin but thick skin similar to that on the forehead or the temple. If the texture of this skin is not eyelid skin, this portion of the "upper eyelid" should be peeled with the Baker's formula rather than with full-strength phenol. If the peel is going to be taped or occluded, the occlusion should include this area below the lateral edge of the upper eyebrow.

Once the entire face has been covered with the Baker's formula, if this is to be an occluded peel, the taping can start. Some physicians start on the forehead and others on the chin. Some use Micropore tape, whereas others use Johnson & Johnson cloth tape (Plate I–I). We are not sure that there is a significant difference. Certainly there has been no proved difference in the various occlusive techniques. Why occlusion works is not known, but it is generally known that occlusion causes greater penetration or efficacy of whatever chemical is being applied percutaneously. With steroid creams, it has been proved that occlusion increases absorption. Exactly what the mechanism is in peeling is not documented. It has been documented that the use of occlusion or a tape mask increases the depth of the wound and, consequently, increases the ability to remove or to correct actinic damage. Some experienced peelers believe that equally good results can be obtained without occlusion. Having watched these physicians, we feel they apply more of the peeling agent than we do, which probably accounts for why we seem to obtain equally satisfactory results.

The mask does not need to be over the entire face or the entire peeled area. It can be applied selectively in those areas that have more sun damage than others. There is nothing wrong with doing a Baker's phenol peel over the entire face and taping only the lower one-third or one-half or the perioral area, leaving the rest open. During the first few weeks of healing, there will be a difference in the amount of crusting and erythema between the open and closed areas. However, within a few months there will be no residual tracks. One of the problems with occlusion in the perioral region is that if the tape becomes macerated from saliva or becomes loosened from movement of the mouth, the effects will be irregular around that area. If the perioral creases are extremely deep, we may dermabrade the perioral cosmetic unit, carrying the abrasion into the lips and into the oral commissures.

It is important to lay the first layers of tape down evenly, with no wrinkles in it. The tape can be 1 inch or ½-inch wide and of whatever length is appropriate to build the mask step by step, strip by strip. There is nothing magic about one, two, or three layers, nor is there any special method that is more effective than another. Along the margin of the mandible, we like to apply the mask in a scissors-like or sawtooth-like fashion so that an irregular line is created at the mandibular margin (Plate II–A). As is well known in cosmetic work, an irregular line is less easily noticed, and thus there is not the sharp contrast between the occluded and unoccluded skin along the mandibular margin. We also use the sawtooth effect around the medial cheek when the entire face is not occluded.

There have been some complications with hypertrophic scarring after phenol peeling, particularly along the mandibular margin and periorally. Some physicians will not tape in these regions because of this incidence of hypertrophic scarring. On the other hand, the radial rhitides around the lips are one of the most common indications for peeling. In these areas of heavy actinic damage, an unoccluded peel is less effective in erasing these wrinkles. In some patients, we have quite successfully taped up to the vermilion border without problems; in other patients, we have seen a development of hypertrophic scarring even when the peel was left unoccluded. It is difficult to advise just what is the best procedure in this perioral area. It seems prudent that, if the patient has had no other procedures in the past, such as dermabrasion, face-lifts, or previous peels, the first peel should be done as deeply as possible because that is the time when there will be the least chance of hypertrophic scarring.

The mask can be left on for 24 or 48 hours. There have been opinions but not evidence in the literature to suggest that one is more effective than the other. In animal studies (by S.J.S., unpublished) there was no difference in the depths of the wounds in the 24-hour vs. the 48-hour occluded peels. The patient is extremely uncomfortable with the tape mask in place, and most are quite happy to take if off. The tape is somewhat painful to remove. The pain certainly is no more intense than that when removing tape from any skin. If there is fine lanugo hair or if the tape has been placed over some of the terminal hairs at the edge of the face, the removal will be more painful. The appearance of the swelling and oozing face often is assumed to be sore; however, we routinely do not give Valium or Demerol before removal of the tape.

After removing the tape, the skin is grayish and edematous, with some areas of desquamation of the damaged epidermis. The entire face is massively edematous, with lips protruding, sometimes everting; eyelids swollen shut; and a generalized serous ooze (Plate II–B). This quite frightening appearance must be explained to the patient and the patient's family before the peel, to minimize anxiety. Regardless of how much preoperative explanation is provided, most people are not prepared to see themselves in this condition.

There are various ways to conduct postoperative care. We are not advocates of creating a thick crust over the peeled area with thymol iodide or other powders. We generally have the patient wash the face in the shower and then use an antibiotic ointment for a few days and then switch to an antibiotic anti-inflammatory cream. The softer the patient keeps the crusts, the less heaped up and irritating they become. We have seen some patients who are loath to touch the face and develop a thick crust over the entire face. We have not seen any evidence that the final result is better whether or not the crust is allowed to form. However, we believe that there is less chance of infection if the wound is kept nearly crust-free and strongly advise using an antibiotic ointment to keep the incidence of *Pseudomonas* surface colonization down.

We have not seen any patients whose scabs required more than two weeks to fall off; actually, the average is seven to ten days. We have heard of patients who need months to heal, but have not had an opportunity to study whether these patients had some inherent metabolic problem. Prior x-ray therapy and long-term corticosteroid therapy can delay healing. We peeled one patient who had a 2-cm area of radiodermatitis on the cheek. That area took three times as long as the surrounding skin to heal, but eventually did so with no problem and with an equally good result.

Makeup can be applied over the skin as soon as the scabs are off. This makeup can be ordinary makeup that is cleansed each day or it can be professional makeup specially designed to help blend out the erythema and the margins between the peeled and unpeeled skin (see chap. 15).

Complete healing requires from three to six months, but the patient's face often is completely acceptable for public appearance without makeup after 30 days. Occasionally there is a prolonged erythema from a chemical peel. This can be a problem for a male but not as much of a problem for a female, who can use makeup. Part of the preoperative consultation should include the information that makeup may be necessary for a period after the peel. If there will be an alteration of the pigmentation, it begins to become visible between three weeks and three months. We usually see hypopigmentation after peels, but there certainly are examples in our own practice and in the literature of hyperpigmentation. If this hyperpigmentation develops, generally it is resistant to most therapy except repeated peel. The second peel, to remove hyperpigmentation, is usually an unoccluded phenol peel or a Baker's formula peel and carries a high rate of success. However, this hyperpigmentation is a complication that one does not like to see. It creates much anxiety for the patient. A re-peel after an appropriate six-month period usually is successful.

For reasons that can only be surmised, the neck does not respond well to treatment, is slower to heal, and tends to have more complications with pigmentary changes and a higher incidence of scarring. Consequently, the neck is seldom peeled. On the other hand, we know of reliable physicians who obtained good results routinely peeling the neck with trichloroacetic acid or a less penetrating phenol procedure. We generally discourage our patients from having the neck peeled, but probably could be talked into it. (Four cases of phenol peeling are shown in Plate II–C to H and on the cover.)

FRESHENING PEELS

We use 35% to 50% trichloroacetic acid peels to treat mild sun damage, light crosshatch wrinkling, and the muddy, irregular pigmentations often found at the end of a long summer of exposure to the sun.[15, 16] The wounds created by 35% to 50% trichloroacetic acid are superficial in comparison to the Baker's formula phenol peel, either occluded or unoccluded, but are as deep a wound as is needed for very early sun damage changes in the upper levels of the dermis.[7, 17]

The technique for these freshening peels is similar to that of the Baker's formula phenol peel except that the entire procedure is done more quickly, is less painful, and less time is required for healing. Preoperative medications, patient preparation, and the application of the agent with one to three cotton-tipped applicators are similar. The frosting, however, is not as quick to appear or as deep in its whitish color. If a great deal of thickened stratum corneum is visible, we increase the strength of the trichloroacetic acid up to 50% to obtain frosting.

Exophytic keratotic lesions, such as seborrheic keratosis, will frost only slightly or not at all. The stratum corneum of these lesions can be disrupted by friction with the wooden end of an applicator stick and then re-treated with trichloroacetic acid to obtain good frosting.

The wound produced by chemical peels is dose-dependent. The amount of the peeling agent can be varied depending on the texture of the skin, with thicker skin receiving more agent than thinner skin. The greater amount of sun damage that one is trying to treat and the more fine crosshatched wrinkling present, the greater the amount of agent that must be used. Using the smallest effective dose, however, always is a good medical principle. This certainly is true with peeling. There is no reason why the different peeling agents cannot be used concurrently. Since the forehead may have little sun damage owing to the protection afforded by hats, the lower half of the face may need a full-strength phenol peel, whereas the forehead can be treated satisfactorily with 30% to 50% trichloroacetic acid.

For these lighter freshening peels, we use just 20% trichloroacetic acid on the eyelids. The application is done in exactly the same way as described previously for the phenol application.

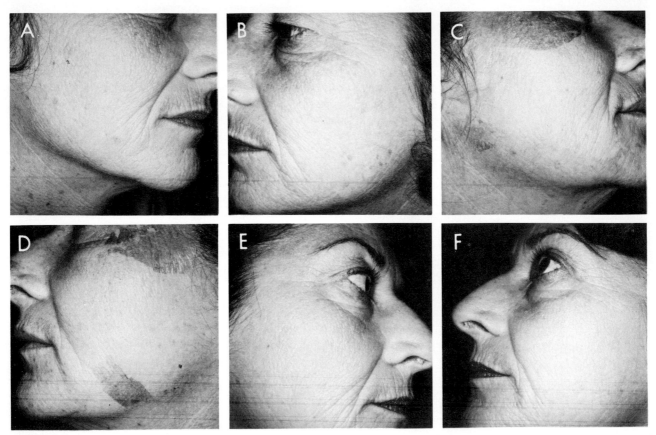

Fig 3–6, A and B.—This 45-year-old woman was treated with a 50% trichloroacetic acid peel to correct the early actinic damage. **C and D,** light crusts and desquamating at five days after the peel. **E and F,** results two months after the procedure.

We do not tape for the freshening peels. Postoperatively, the patient is given the same medications discussed above, daily showers, plus an antibiotic ointment for the first few days, followed by anti-inflammatory antibiotic cream. Healing is much quicker with the more superficial wound. Some patients develop a fine, even crusting within 3 to 5 days, which is shed completely in 7 days. Whereas we may tell patients who have an occluded phenol peel that we expect them to be completely out of the public's eye for a minimum of 14 days, patients who have the freshening peel may be back to work after 7 days, with a light cover makeup to counteract the pinkness and erythema of the freshly peeled skin.

It is our observation, but not in any way proved, that postinflammatory hyperpigmentation is more common after some of these light peels. The patient will look pink and beautiful at 10 to 14 days, and by 30 to 45 days have a surprisingly dark brownish mask at the peeled area. In our experience, this hyperpigmentation always has faded, but it can be a disconcerting and troublesome interlude. We generally treat this hyperpigmentation with one of the bleaching formulas. However, we are not sure that these bleach creams do anything in addition to the natural resolution of postinflammatory hyperpigmentation (Fig 3–6).

50% TRICHLOROACETIC ACID, OCCLUDED PEEL

Many physicians believe that it is not safe to use phenol preparations for face peeling. To avoid using the phenol peel while trying to achieve good treatment for sun-damaged skin and wrinkling, they use the maximum nonscarring level of trichloroacetic acid, which is 50% to 60%, and may occlude in the standard way with tape. There is no doubt from our clinical experience and from histologic studies that occlusion of 50% trichloroacetic acid enhances the depth of the wound and thus, we believe, the cosmetic improvement.

The preoperative procedure, the application of the trichloroacetic acid, the taping, and postsurgical follow-up all are quite similar, if not exactly as described for the occluded Baker's formula phenol mixture. Healing is somewhat more rapid than with the occluded phenol mixture, and there is less edema. Actually, the discomfort of removing the tape on the first or second day is somewhat increased since the tape does not tend to "float off" with the serum exudate as much as it does after a phenol peel. The entire procedure is not quite as severe, since the crusting period is shorter, the postoperative erythema is of shorter duration, and, unfortunately, the depth of the peel is not such that it removes the deeper wrinkles.

This technique is acceptable for moderate sun damage and moderate wrinkling, particularly on the cheeks, forehead, and lateral canthal area. However, it is not particularly effective for the perioral rhitides. We have several patients who have had a beautiful result after trichloroacetic acid occluded peel but no significant improvement in the perioral creases and wrinkles. The complaint that lipstick would run into these creases still was present after the trichloroacetic acid occluded peel. The results are not as predictably good from trichloroacetic acid peels as from phenol peels.

FULL STRENGTH PHENOL UN-OCCLUDED PEEL

In our hands, the open, full-strength phenol peel has results similar to but more dependable than those of the occluded 50%–60% trichloroacetic acid peel. The technique is simpler in that the tape is not used. Therefore, the discomfort from the tape, the need for the second visit, and the added discomfort of removing the tape all are avoided. This technique is particularly favored by cosmetic surgeons to freshen the skin after a rhytidectomy (three to six months) for that patient who does not have severe wrinkles or perioral creases. From our experience, we believe that the full-strength, open phenol peel and the 50% to 60% trichloroacetic acid peel, occluded or un-occluded, yield very similar results. However, for moderate to severe aging changes, the result of an open trichloroacetic acid peel is most unpredictable. Too often the depth of the wound is variable and the correction is splotchy.

PIGMENTARY CHANGES

One of the most frequent and bothersome side effects of use of any peeling agent is unpredictable changes in pigmentation.[18–21] Clearly, phenol is toxic to the melanocytes, and some lightening or hypopigmentation can be expected after its use. This change, however, is not universal or predictable. We have seen cases in our own practice and in others in which a permanent hyperpigmentation resulted after a peel.

The effect of phenol or trichloroacetic acid on pigmented lesions, such as lentigines and seborrheic keratoses, also is unpredictable. We certainly have seen cases in which such hyperpigmented lesions faded with the phenol and thus were erased. Intradermal nevi often get darker, and freckles tend to be erased with these procedures. However, we have also seen cases where the skin surrounding a lentigo was lightened so that the hyperpigmented lesion became more obvious. Seborrheic keratoses can be removed by peeling as described in chapter 2. There is less hypopigmentation after the use of trichloroacetic acid; however, as mentioned earlier, the incidence of temporary hyperpigmentation seems to be higher.

It is essential to discuss these possibilities with the patient before treatment. The porcelain appearance of skin, severely hypopigmented and smooth skin resulting from a full-face occluded phenol peel is attractive on some patients but a terrible problem for people who are not fair-complexioned. The dividing line between the peeled and unpeeled areas of the face or neck is much more obvious in patients with darker coloring. Any cosmetic surgeon likes to see the blue-eyed, blond-haired, and fair-complexioned patient because this skin does not show tracks so obviously. Next to this patient, we like to see the woman who habitually wears complete foundation makeup because she, too, can cover our tracks.

We use bleaching agents such as 6% hydroquinone in vehicle-N; Melanex; and the combination of 3% hydroquinone, 0.1% triamcinolone acetonide, and 0.1% retinoic acid, but we are not sure how truly effective these agents are. In any condition where pigmentation is affected, either hypopigmentation or hyperpigmentation, avoidance of strong sun for three to six months is essential. The sunscreens available today are excellent and come in a wide variety of vehicles. Good patient instruction on the use of a sunscreen, as well as avoidance of the sun, is an essential part of every face peel.

In certain patients and in certain types of aging skin, dermabrasion is just as effective, and there are different potentials for pigmentary changes with dermabrasion (see chap. 4).

OTHER INDICATIONS

We believe that the primary indication for face peeling is sun-damaged skin. Far down the list there are other indications, but we believe that the results from these other indications are so unpredictable that we mention them here only for completeness.

Telangiectasias are not affected in any predictable way by any of the peeling agents.

The size of the pores of the sebaceous area of the face also probably is not affected in any way by a face peel, except that removal of the stratum corneum may make the pores appear more obvious; the change is temporary.

Although there is a variety of postacne scars, none of them, except possibly hyperpigmentation, is significantly affected by any of the peeling agents. Sometimes in the first few months after a peel, when the interstitial edema is present and the collagen healing is continuing in the dermis, some of the depressed scars appear less depressed. This is a temporary phenomenon of edema. Patients often are of the opinion that the peel has reduced their scarring, but they forget how their skin really looked in the six-month interval from the time of the peel until the time it was completely healed.

Melasma is a terrible problem for some patients. All of us in our desperation to try to help them occasionally will try to peel the skin. We think that this is acceptable as long as the patient is fully advised that the procedure is a trial and that results are unpredictable. One of the problems with test spot peels (or dermabrasion, for that matter) is that there is no guarantee that the rest of the skin on the face will respond as did the test spot. We are aware of cases in which peeling agents used for treatment of melasma resulted only in deeper and more extensive melasma.

SCARRING

Fortunately, scarring is an infrequent if persistent complication of face peeling.[18-20] It is tragic when someone comes in seeking an improvement in appearance and leaves with general improvement, but with a localized scar. The most common areas for the development of scarring are in the upper lip area and the angle of the jaw (Fig 3–7). There are many hypotheses as to why these areas scar more. Some physicians believe that movement of the face is contributory and ask their patients to keep the face quiet for several weeks. This always sounds good at meetings or in papers but probably is impractical. One wonders whether those physicians really believe that their patients can keep the face quiet for as long as they would like them to. Dermal healing is most active between 6 and 20 weeks. It is the deep dermal wounds that lead to scarring. Another theory has to do with the thinness of the skin, but one need examine only a few hundred faces to realize that the thickness of the skin varies with every patient and with every portion of the face. If this were truly a factor, we would expect to see scarring on some people in the temples, in others on the jowls, and in still others on the bridge of the nose. If the patient had rhytidectomy with undermining, previous peels, or previous dermabrasions, the incidence of scarring definitely is higher.

We treat this scarring as we do all scarring: with time, support, and cortisone. The cortisone can be used intralesionally (triamcinolone acetonide 4 to 20 mg ml); topically with the strong fluorinated corticosteroids in creams, gels, or ointments, or impregnated into tapes (Cordran tape).

Some physicians will not tape-occlude the angle of the mandible or the upper lip. This, of course, will reduce the incidence of scarring. However, the upper lip area is one of the most prominent areas of the face. This wrinkling

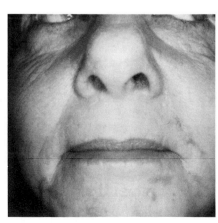

Fig 3–7.—Eight weeks after a full-strength phenol occluded peel showing the development of indurated scaling in the perioral and chin areas.

of the perioral region is what brings many women to us for improvement so that it is difficult not to recommend taping the upper lip. But we believe that the risk must be explained to the patient, since that area, more than all others, must be treated with the deepest possible wounding to obtain the best results. We do tape the upper lip and tape it onto the vermilion border to remove the wrinkles at the upper portion of the vermilion. (For the same reason, we also dermabrade onto the vermilion.) However, the results of peeling are not as predictably good around the mouth as with dermabrasion, in which the physician has absolute control of the depth of the wound. Also, it is unlikely that the tape of the occluded peel remains tightly sealed around the mouth.

CONCLUSION

After reading this chapter, it would be entirely understandable for physicians who do not do peels to believe that peels are not worth the risk to the patient or the efforts of the physician. This is an understandable feeling. The main motivation for doing peels is that they work—patients who have prematurely aging skin again can have normal skin for their peer group; patients who have other cosmetic surgery now can have beautiful, fresh-appearing skin on their new contour lines; and patients who do not have other cosmetic surgery but who look ill and dull again can have a radiant complexion. This is one of the most rewarding of all cosmetic procedures but also one that requires a great deal of support for the patient.

Another conclusion from reading this chapter might be that one should not do the procedure without having observed an experienced physician performing the technique. There is so much nonscience involved in face peeling that the technique can be passed only from operator to operator, with each physician being careful not to assume that there is only one way to achieve good results. It is hoped that in time, more scientific studies can be undertaken, and dose-response curves, estimates of the thickness of the damaged skin vs. the amount of escharotic agent needed, and safety parameters all can be outlined to make the procedure more appealing for more patients to undergo and for more physicians to perform.

REFERENCES

1. Baker T.J., Gordon H.L.: The ablation of rhitides by chemical means, a preliminary report. *J. Fla. Med. Assoc.* 48:451, 1961.
2. Baker T.J.: Chemical face peeling and rhytidectomy. *Plast. Reconstr. Surg.* 29:199, 1962.
3. Baker T.J., Gordon H.L.: Chemosurgery of the face, some warnings and misconceptions. *J. Fla. Med. Assoc.* 49:218, 1962.
4. Baker T.J., Gordon H.L.: Chemical face peeling, an adjunct to surgical face lifting. *South Med. J.* 56:412, 1963.
5. Baker T.J., Gordon H.L., Seckinger D.L.: A second look at chemical face peeling. *Plast. Reconstr. Surg.* 37:487, 1966.
6. Mosienko P., Baker T.J.: Chemical peel. *Clin. Plast. Surg.* 5:1, 1978
7. Stegman S.J.: Histologic changes on normal and sundamaged skin produced by various chemical peeling agents. *Aesth. Plast. Surg.* 6:123-135, 1982.
8. Harkness R.A., Beveridge G.W., Davidson D.W.: Percutaneous absorption of *l*-naphthol-(^{14}C) in man. *Br. J. Dermatol.* 85:49, 1971.
9. Conning D.M., Hayes M.J.: The dermal toxicity of phenol: an investigation of the most effective first-aid measures. *Br. J. Ind. Med.* 27:155-159, 1970.

10. Spira M., Dahl C., Freeman R., et al.: Chemosurgery—a histological study. *Plast. Reconstr. Surg.* 45:247-253, 1970.
11. Brown V.K.H., Box V.L., Simpson B.J.: Decontamination procedures for skin exposed to phenolic substances. *Arch. Environ. Health* 30:1-6, 1975.
12. Baker T.J., Gordon H.L.: Chemical face peeling and dermabrasion. *Surg. Clin. North Am.* 51:387-401, 1971.
13. Baker T.J., Gordon H.L., Mosienko P., et al.: Long-term histological study of skin after chemical face peeling. *Plast. Reconstr. Surg.* 53:522-525, 1974.
14. Truppman E.S., Ellenberg J.D.: Major electrocardiographic changes during chemical face peeling. *Plast Reconstr. Surg.* 63:44, 1979.
15. Resnik S.S., Lewis L.A., Cohen B.H.: Trichloroacetic acid peeling. *Cutis* 17:127-129, 1976.
16. Resnik S.S., Lewis L.A.: The cosmetic uses of trichloroacetic acid peeling in dermatology. *South. Med. J.* 66:225, 1973.
17. Behin F., Feuerstein S.S., Marovitz W.F.: Comparative histological study of mini pig skin after chemical peel and dermabrasion. *Arch. Otolaryngol.* 103:271-277, 1977.
18. Litton C., Trinidad G.: Complications of chemical face peeling as evaluated by a questionnaire. *Plast. Reconstr. Surg.* 67:738-743, 1981.
19. Spira M., Gerow F.J., Hardy S.B.: Complications of chemical face peeling. *Plast. Reconstr. Surg.* 54:397-403, 1974.
20. Aronsohn R.B.: Complications of chemosurgery. *Eye, Ear, Nose, Throat Monthly,* January 1972.
21. Lotter A.M.: Human pigment factors relative to chemical face peeling. *Ann. Plast. Surg.* 3:231-240, 1979.

4 / Dermabrasion Equipment

THERE IS A variety of machines, dermabrading tips, and techniques used for dermabrasion. There are strong advocates of each tool or technique, but we find that although different approaches provide specific benefits for individual operators, they seldom alter the results. Equally good results (Fig 4–1) are obtainable with all of the techniques described below unless stated otherwise. How each operator utilizes the tools determines the result.

Although dermabrasion can be done with hand units, almost all operators use a power source that is either electrical or compressed nitrogen gas. In general, compressed nitrogen provides greater torque and faster revolutions. However, the inconvenience of having to store, chain to the wall, and replace nitrogen tanks leads most operators to use the electrical motors.

The standard for many years was the cable-driven type in which the motor rotated a cable approximately 4 ft long. The rotating cable then turned the dermabrading end-piece. This mechanism was typified by the Robbins unit (Fig 4–2), which provides rotation speeds of 800–12,000 rpm. Hundreds of thousands of dermabrasions were successfully done with this type of apparatus. In using cable-driven machines, the operator must be sure that the cable is kept straight or in no more than a very gentle curve. Sharp bends on the

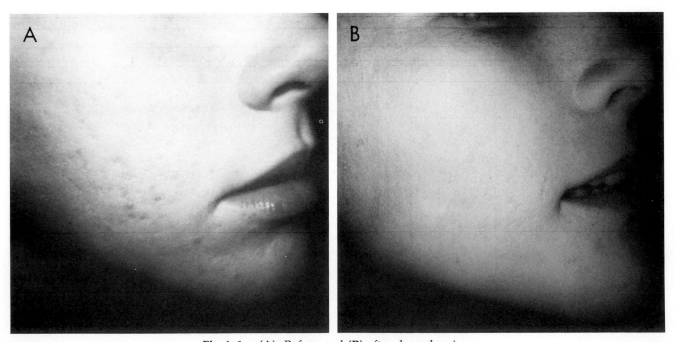

Fig 4–1.—(A), Before and **(B)** after dermabrasion.

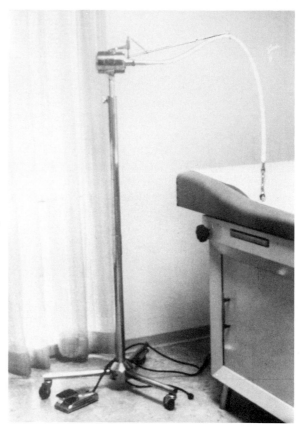

Fig 4–2.—Cable-driven dermabrader, Robbins type.

cable create excess friction, resulting in a burnout of the cable. In addition, the cable apparatus emits a high-speed whine that is inherently more distressing to the patient and to the physician than the nitrogen-driven machines or the new hand engines.

The nitrogen-driven machines typified by the Stryker apparatus are used predominantly by plastic surgeons and only rarely by dermatologists. This differential most likely is based on the fact that plastic surgeons still perform many dermabrasions in the hospital, where this equipment is available. Also, certain companies tend to sell their products predominantly to practitioners of certain specialties.

In the past ten years, advances in technology have led to the making of small electrical engines that can be held in the hand (Fig 4–3,A). These are attached to electronic controls by a simple, coiled cord that permits maximal flexibility for operator use. These are typified by the Bell hand engine, Model 5-B,* which rotates at 400–16,000 rpm, and faster units such as the Model 8-A,† which provides 600–33,000 rpm (Fig 4–3,B). These machines are supposed to provide torque compensation so that torque is maintained at 80% of normal. However, in clinical use, the torque available from these machines is less than that provided by other types, although still adequate for dermabrasion. It is the com-

---

*Model 5-B replaced by 25D (speed: crawl to 18,000 rpm).
†Model 8-AL replaced by 28L (speed: 2,000–35,000 rpm).

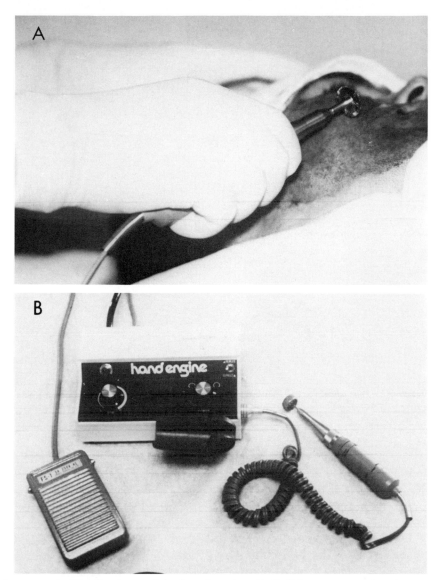

Fig 4–3.—A, Hand grip used for hand engine. **B,** Bell International hand engine.

bination of speed and torque that provides the rapid cutting desired. Some machines will rotate up to 125,000 rpm but have so little torque that they barely turn when applied to the skin. The hand engines now are our favorite machines for dermabrasion.

The dermabrasion equipment with the greatest speed and torque is typified by the high-speed Schreuss (Derma III) machine, manufactured by A. Schumann Precision Manufacturer, Dusseldorf, but available both in the United States and Germany.‡ This unit rotates at 15,000–60,000 rpm and retains a strong torque. Only a few of these machines are in use in the United States.

---

‡A. Schumann Precision Manufacturers, Concord, Mass.

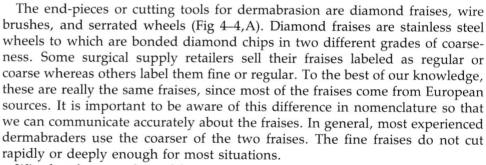

Fig 4–4.—A, Types of dermabrasion tips used: *left,* serrated wheel; *right,* wire brush; rest are diamond fraises. **B,** Kurtin wire brush showing individual wire construction. **C,** Serrated wheel showing stainless steel teeth.

The end-pieces or cutting tools for dermabrasion are diamond fraises, wire brushes, and serrated wheels (Fig 4–4,A). Diamond fraises are stainless steel wheels to which are bonded diamond chips in two different grades of coarseness. Some surgical supply retailers sell their fraises labeled as regular or coarse whereas others label them fine or regular. To the best of our knowledge, these are really the same fraises, since most of the fraises come from European sources. It is important to be aware of this difference in nomenclature so that we can communicate accurately about the fraises. In general, most experienced dermabraders use the coarser of the two fraises. The fine fraises do not cut rapidly or deeply enough for most situations.

Wire brushes are claimed by some operators to be the superior end-piece. The wire brush developed by Abner Kurtin and Noel Robbins and was the earliest successful dermabrasion end-piece used in modern times. Therefore, if you learned dermabrasion in the 1950s and 1960s, you probably learned with the Kurtin wire brush. The earliest students, who naturally became the national spokesmen, then touted with great praise the Kurtin wire brush as the only way to do a good dermabrasion

This brush is a stainless steel wheel with wires arranged at an angle, as shown in Figure 4–4,B. The wires of the brush cut deeply and rapidly in frozen skin. The tiny pieces of tissue cut out by the brush are thrown away from the operating field by centrifugal force. In contrast, there is another type of wire brush that seldom is mentioned, a contra-angled or right-angle brush. Here, the ends of the wires act in a manner more like brushes in a street cleaner or an electrical car polisher. In contrast to the Kurtin wire brush, which cuts deeply and rapidly, the contra-angled brush takes off quite thin pieces of tissue and does not throw as many from the field. Many are retained in the operative field mixed with blood, a paste of slurry is created. We mention this contra-angled wire brush only for completeness, but do not recommend it.

Serrated wheels represent an attempt to obtain the benefits of both the diamond fraise and the wire brush. These are stainless steel wheels with rows of sharp points projecting from the surface (Fig 4–4,C). By applying pressure, serrated wheels can cut deeply and rapidly, but with light pressure have an action similar to that of the diamond fraise.

CARE OF EQUIPMENT

It is important to have standard care of dermabrasion equipment. Bell hand engines may need to be lubricated after every few uses according to the manufacturer's instructions. Cable-driven equipment should be maintained so that the cables always are clean and rotate freely. If any unusual noises are heard from the engines, repair requests should be made immediately. There always should be a backup system no matter which system is used. We like the simple Dremel hobby Moto-tool (Fig 4–5). Our office has performed a number of full-face dermabrasions with the various Dremel tools. The speed and torque are excellent. However, the unpleasant high-speed whine is a great deterrent to standard use of this inexpensive machine. If some company could make a hobby tool with a more pleasant sound, it could quickly capture a share of the dermabrasion machine market. We had a plastic surgeon neighbor who did not heed this backup rule, but we were able to loan him our backup Dremel

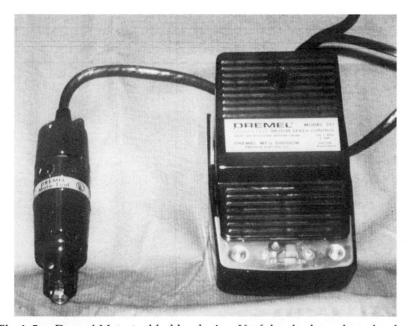

Fig 4–5.—Dremel Moto-tool hobby device. Useful as back-up dermabrader.

machine so that he could complete the second half of his dermabrasion after his expensive machine broke down in the middle of the procedure.

Dermabrasion tips also must be maintained in good order. They should be washed thoroughly with a nylon surgical hand brush, detergent, and elbow grease. Electronic cleaning devices have proved to be less effective for us. Kurtin brushes need a special wire combing hand device to clean blood and debris that gathers between the wires of the brush.

The end-pieces then are packaged and sterilized in the autoclave. Diamond fraises wear with repeated use, as do wire brushes. Examine the tips to be sure that the cutting edge is still good. Wire brushes will lose their effectiveness quicker than the serrated wheel or the diamond fraise. Hold the shaft in your fingers and twirl the end-piece so that it runs against your fingers. In this way you can feel whether the brushes are worn and need replacement. Sometimes the brushes are good for only a few dermabrasions and will require periodic replacement.

A PRACTICE MODEL

When trying out a new dermabrasion technique, such as those described below, it is best first to try the technique on a grapefruit. The grapefruit represents the single best laboratory demonstration for practice with the diamond fraise because you can relate changes in the grapefruit's skin to those that occur in human skin. As you initially dermabrade the grapefruit, the yellow color is removed, revealing a white skin below (Fig 4–6,A). This is equivalent to removing the human epidermis with its pigment layer. Slightly deeper dermabrasion becomes analogous to being at the level of the papillary dermis in human skin, where the holes or pores of the grapefruit, analogous to the sebaceous glands, begin to show more prominently (Fig 4–6,B). As these holes appear larger, the depth is equivalent to the upper dermal layers in human skin (Fig 4–6,C). As you abrade even more deeply, there are fewer and smaller pores in the grapefruit's skin, analogous to the lower reticular dermis, where most sebaceous glands have disappeared (Fig 4–6,D). The next dermabrasion level on the grapefruit skin reveals purple, darker areas. You now have gone through the outer skin of the grapefruit into the pulp (Fig 4–6,E). This is analogous to going through human skin and seeing the yellow fat globules indicating the subcutaneous depth.

By practicing on the grapefruit with the diamond fraise and relating it to the human skin, you can visualize the approximate depth of your dermabrasion and, therefore, more accurately select the amount of wound you desire. Using the diamond fraise, the levels of dermabrasion on human skin can be determined readily. They are introduced at this point to reinforce the importance of knowing the levels and making the practice on grapefruit meaningful for later work on humans (Fig 4–7).

In human facial skin, level 1 is reached when there is a change to a lighter color, indicating that the epidermis with its melanocytes has been removed. Also, tiny vessels of the subepidermal plexus are seen. Level 2 is reached when these tiny vessels disappear and tiny yellow dots are just perceived. This indicates that most or all of the papillary dermis has been removed, the yellow dots representing the tops of sebaceous glands seen through some remaining dermal collagen fibers. Level 3 is reached when larger and more numerous

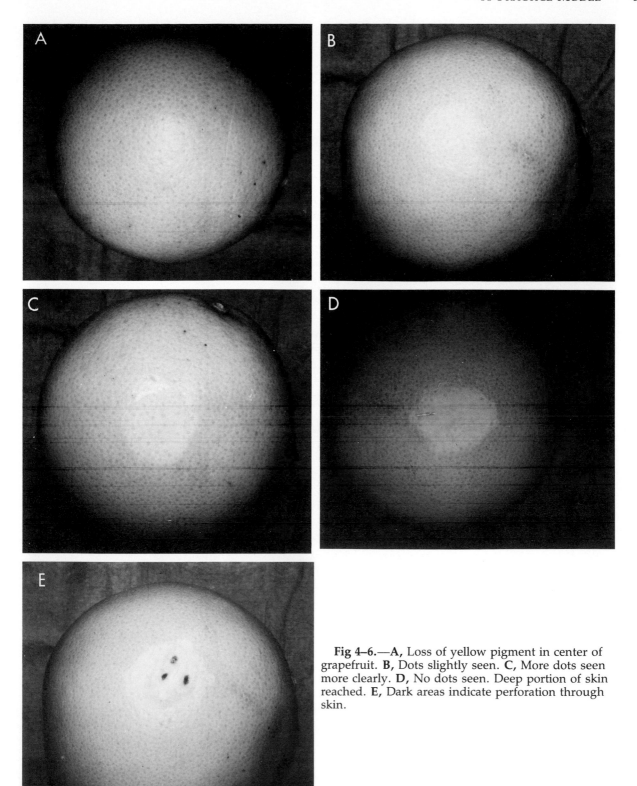

Fig 4–6.—**A,** Loss of yellow pigment in center of grapefruit. **B,** Dots slightly seen. **C,** More dots seen more clearly. **D,** No dots seen. Deep portion of skin reached. **E,** Dark areas indicate perforation through skin.

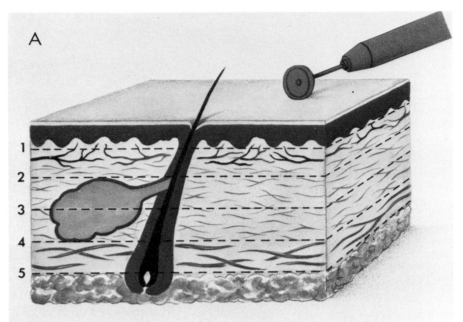

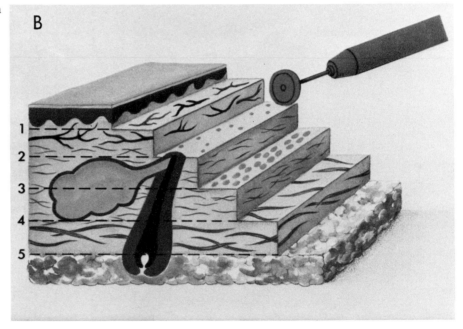

Fig 4–7.—A, The five levels of dermabrasion. **B,** Stepwise demonstration of the structures seen at the five levels of dermabrasion.

yellow dots are seen, indicating that the middle of the sebaceous glands has been reached, which is essentially the mid-dermis. Level 4 is reached when the larger yellow dots become smaller and fewer or totally disappear. This plane is the deeper reticular dermis. Level 5 is reached when very large yellow globules are seen, indicating invasion completely through the skin into the subcutaneous layer. In practice, level 5 should *never* be reached. If it is accidently reached, the area of abrasion through the skin should be sutured with 6-0 or 5-0 Vicryl and Dexon to reestablish dermal continuity. Left unsutured, level 5 dermabraded areas generally result in hypertrophic scars. Memorize the five levels of dermabrading human skin with the diamond fraise and think of them as you practice on your grapefruit so that during your first human dermabrasion you know how deep you are at all times. When doing dermabrasions on human skin, record the level(s) of dermabrasion reached so that you can more accurately compare your own work among your patients and more scientifically compare your dermabrasion successes and problems with other physicians who use the five-level system.

These levels of dermabrasion do not show on human skin when using the wire brush, but show quite well with the diamond fraise. For wire brush practice, a fresh pig's foot and Freon spray are best. Notice the character and fraying of the collagen fibers. In human skin, fraying of coarse collagen fibers is the end point of dermabrasion.

PREOPERATIVE STUDIES

Preoperative blood work on dermabrasion patients varies with each physician. Some prefer to take a complete medical history and do only a test-spot dermabrasion. For them, this provides the needed information regarding bleeding and clotting, healing, and pigmentary changes. Test spots usually are oval or rectangular and placed along the hairline of the temple or in the preauricular region. If the patient does not then have a full dermabrasion or if, for some reason, the physician discovers some untoward effects and does not recommend further dermabrasion, this small area of skin is hardly noticeable.

Other physicians prefer to obtain a complete blood cell count, SMA panel, and bleeding and clotting panels. Other physicians will obtain the above-mentioned laboratory work as well as a hepatitis panel. If there is evidence of hepatitis antibody or high hepatitis antigen levels, some physicians will not perform the surgery. There are cases of physicians and their staff having contracted hepatitis from patients while doing dermabrasion.

All three of these groups of physicians are "performing good medical care." One must choose which is the correct approach for his own practice.

PREOPERATIVE MEDICATION

A variety of approaches is used for preoperative medications. Historically, 50–100 mg of Demerol IM, with 25 mg of Phenergan, was favored. The Phenergan was given on the mistaken premise that it enhances the analgesic effect of Demerol. A Compazine-Demerol combination now is favored by some in the belief that Compazine reduces the nausea caused by Demerol.

Valium 5–10 mg given IV slowly over several minutes is a sedative commonly used by cosmetic surgeons who have an open IV line and are in a hospital operating room or a fully equipped office surgery. The Valium can be titrated throughout the procedure; IM Valium also can be used. However, rarely a patient may have apnea from IV Valium and require intubation. We, too, like Valium; however, we prefer the following approach: 10 mg of Valium is given orally and 50–100 mg of Demerol is given IM 30 minutes before the procedure. An additional 5–10 mg of Valium is given sublingually. As the patient lets the Valium dissolve under the tongue, relaxation ensues within 15–20 minutes without significant untoward side effects. This gains rapid tranquilization while waiting for the oral dose to become effective. Further relaxation and relief from pain can be provided by 50 mg of Demerol given later in the operation. Within the first hour after the dermabrasion, there is a lot of stinging of the entire dermabraded area. Demerol given later in the procedure helps to relieve this pain until the patient can get home, into bed, and take codeine orally.

It should be pointed out that sublingual Valium has not been approved by the FDA. We have used it for more than five years in our practice and find it safe and effective, without untoward side effects.

General anesthesia is favored by a small number of dermatologists and by more cosmetic surgeons who are accustomed to using the hospital operatory. There is no question that general anesthesia provides for easier, more rapid dermabrasion and is far less stressful for the patient and the surgeon. We enjoy doing dermabrasions even more when the patient has general anesthesia. However, we use it only in rare cases; e.g., teenagers who are not able to cooperate, mentally deficient people, and the rare patient who absolutely cannot tolerate discomfort. Because of the occasional idiosyncratic reaction and a few anesthesia-related deaths and, more important, because most people tolerate the procedure well without general anesthesia, we seldom recommend its routine use.

Other combinations, nitrous oxide, low-dose IV Demerol, and Penthrane whistles, have been described and are valuable in certain circumstances. We find that Valium given orally and sublingually is the easiest for office procedures.

LOCAL ANESTHESIA

Nerve blocks to the major facial nerves with Xylocaine, Duranest, or Marcaine often are used. The technique includes a direct nerve block of the infraor-

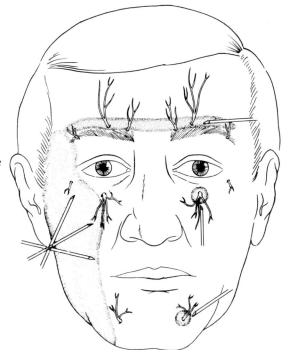

Fig 4–8.—Technique of nerve blocks and local infiltration to locally anesthetize 95% of the face.

bital and mental nerves. The supraorbital, supratrochlear, and temporofacial nerves are blocked by a line of anesthesia infiltrated from the lateral edge of one eyebrow to the lateral edge of the other. The temporozygomatic nerves emerging from their foramina are blocked by field infiltration of the lateral malar area. With the cooperative patient, the whole central cheek also can be infiltrated locally. These injections provide anesthesia for 95% of the face with only about 25 ml of solution (Fig 4–8). The patient then has a minimum of pain during the procedure, and if the long-lasting anesthetic agents are used, most of the postoperative discomfort is avoided. We have been using local anesthetics for five years in our office and are quite happy with the results. Doing so makes the entire procedure easier for the physician and for the patient.

PROPHYLACTIC ANTIBIOTICS

Prophylactic antibiotics are used by many physicians doing dermabrasion. The general rule is that the antibiotic should be in the tissue before the physician. Some physicians inject one dose of cephalosporin along with premedications; others give oral erythromycin, tetracycline, or semisynthetic penicillins before the procedure and continue for one, two, or seven days after the dermabrasion. The consensus indicates that the antibiotic is effective if given up to two to four hours following the procedure. Obviously, to have the antibiotic in the tissue prior to the operation is favored. The need for prophylactic antibiotics in dermabrasion is doubtful. It may be that they have more of a psychological and medicolegal value than a scientific one. Nevertheless, each physician must determine for himself whether he believes that prophylactic antibiotics should be given.

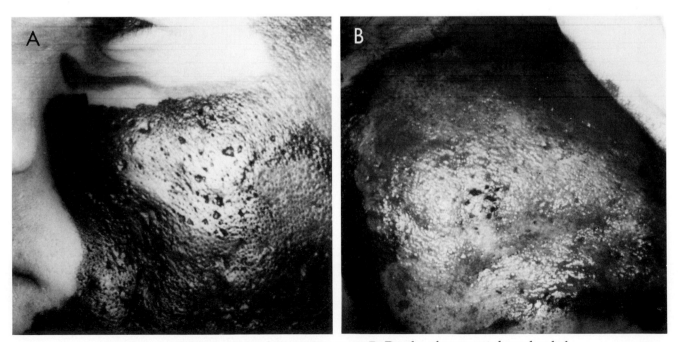

Fig 4–9.—**A,** Gentian violet demarcating scars. **B,** Depths of scars not dermabraded. These will require individual attention with the bullet fraise.

GENERAL TECHNIQUE

Some physicians pre-cool the face with ice packs or cold polyglycol gel bags for 10–15 minutes prior to dermabrasion. This technique is helpful but not necessary. The patient is positioned lying on the back on a comfortable table without a pillow. It should be possible to turn the patient's face from side to side so that the cheek and temple will represent a flat surface, essentially parallel to the plane of the top of the table.

Aqueous 1% gentian violet applied with cotton applicators often is used and is helpful in two ways. One is to demarcate the limit of the dermabrasion, which is helpful because when the face is bloody and covered with towels, it is not difficult to miss a section that one had planned to dermabrade. Wide lines of gentian violet are drawn at the infraorbital rims and just below the jawline. Gentian violet also is used to paint the depths of the scars (Fig 4–9). Theoretically, when the gentian violet has been dermabraded away from the bottom of the scar, all of that scar has been completely abraded. This is not really what happens. Since the gentian violet is scraped out of the bottom of the scar before the surrounding tissue is abraded to the base of the scar, it does not tell the operator the depth of the dermabrasion. It is helpful, however, to highlight deeper scars.

Although gauze squares commonly are used in dermabrasion, ordinary soft, sterile dishtowels or baby diapers or paper are far superior. Gauze squares occasionally get caught by the whirling tip of the dermabrader, causing a frightening, flapping sound. Catching a gauze square can result in breaking of the cable or serious damage to the bearings of the hand engine. The dermabrasion tip is less likely to become caught on the dishtowel or baby diaper.

Many operators and assistants like to wear cloth gloves because they provide better traction than rubber gloves when working in a wet, bloody field. Some wear sterile surgical gloves beneath the cotton ones to protect them from the

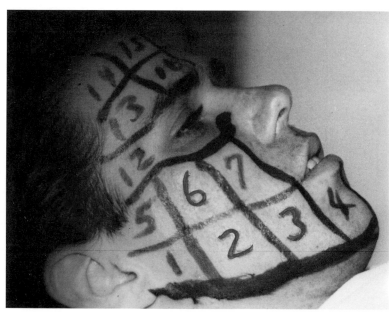

Fig 4–10.—Subdividing and numbering sequential areas for dermabrasion. Allows assistant to know exactly which section you wish to dermabrade next.

blood. The double gloves provide insulation against the cold spray as well as protection from hepatitis. We used cloth gloves for a number of years and found that if we were careful with the way we used the towels or diapers, the rubber gloves worked well and we still were able to gain good traction on the wet, oozing skin. However, there is no doubt that the cotton gloves give a much firmer grasp of the patient's face, although they do not protect against hepatitis when used alone.

Dermabrasion is planned and performed in segments. Some operators mark with gentian violet the various segments on the skin and the order in which they are to be treated (Fig 4–10). Others block off the segments with folded towels (Fig 4–11,A and B). Whichever approach is used, the most dependent portion of the face always is dermabraded first. If a superior area is dermabraded first, the blood tends to run over the area that is going to be abraded, occluding the field. Some operators start in front of the ear and move to the angle of the jaw and to the lateral chin. Others prefer to start on the chin and work in a reverse fashion.

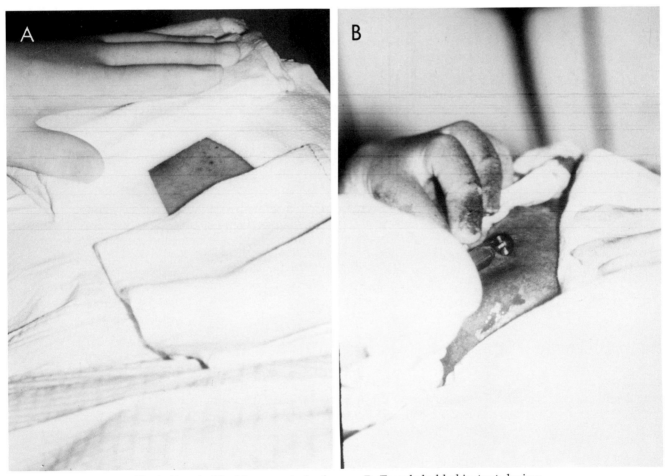

Fig 4–11.—**A,** Blocking area to be frozen. **B,** Towels hold skin taut during dermabrasion and prevent blood from running into the field.

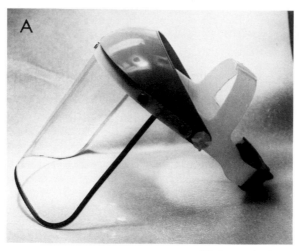
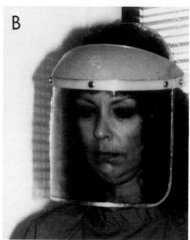
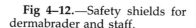
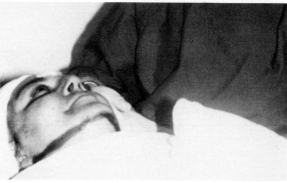

Fig 4–12.—Safety shields for dermabrader and staff.

Cotton should be placed into the ear canals so that freezing material or blood does not pool and disturb the patient. When we are spraying around the nostrils, we try to develop a rhythm with the patient whereby we count to three, during which time the patient takes a deep breath. Then, after three, we spray for a few seconds while the patient holds the breath. Soon, the patient participates in this rhythm and no cryogen is inhaled.

The room should be approximately 62° F so that freezing will take place faster. Also, it is important to have doors or windows open or good ventilation in order to obtain good freezing.

It is best that all operating personnel wear face shields (Fig 4–12,A and B) because the skin and blood splatter. At various times throughout the procedure it will be necessary to wash the surface with soap or detergent to maintain good visibility. Some operators like to use a splatter guard on the dermabrasion machine to catch the splatter. The guard clearly prevents most of the spray from splattering the masks. At the same time, it does block some view of the dermabrasion end-piece. It is a matter of choice for each dermabrader. During dermabrasion, it is absolutely essential that the physician and the assistants at all times keep their eyes on the end-piece when it is in motion and in contact with the skin. By paying such careful attention, mistakes are less likely to be made.

When one side of the cheek and chin is completed, a folded towel is applied to the dermabraded area and the patient's head is turned to the other side. Again, it is important to have a perfectly flat surface to dermabrade. The same sequence of events is followed when doing the chin and forehead and, therefore, the face must be repositioned.

FREEZING TECHNIQUE

There is a great variation in the amount of freezing that different operators desire. Freezing "board hard" is *always* required when using the wire brush. With proper anesthesia, it is possible to dermabrade with the diamond fraise with no freezing at all. It is clear, however, that the harder the freeze, the easier it is to dermabrade deeply. This is not to say that deep dermabrasion cannot be obtained without a hard freeze,[8] but it implies that without it, abrading to the level of the lower dermis, except when using a 60,000-rpm machine, would be difficult. Some physicians freeze lightly only to obtain analgesia when using the diamond fraise.

One measure of the depth of the dermabrasion is the healing time. If all of the scabs are off within five to seven days, it is unlikely that the abrasion extended much below the papillary dermis. If the crusts are off by the third day, the procedure was only "epidermabrasion."

One of us (S. J. S.) has performed histologic studies on guinea pigs to determine the effect of wounding from the freeze alone. Frigiderm spray was used on the backs of guinea pigs after the hair had been removed. The samples taken immediately and at three days clearly showed that a spray of 10 seconds produced almost no wounding, whereas a spray of 20 seconds caused edema of the epidermis and papillary dermis. If 10-second sprays are repeated, allowing complete defrosting between sprays, there still is no wounding. However, a repeated 20-second spray compounds the depth of the wound. These data have not been published.

Although guinea pig skin is different from human skin, certain qualities in response to wounding are the same, and these similarities have been pointed out in a recently published paper.[1] There also are excellent studies for human skin published in the 1950s and 1960s that show that the freezing effect has minimal contribution to the overall wound as produced by dermabrasion.[2-4]

If an extremely hard freeze is desired, two assistants spraying, or one spraying with two cans, will be required. For this degree of freezing, the skin should be hard enough to have a rigid, board-like feeling. The operator signals for the assistant to start the freeze and then signals when he believes that it is frozen to the appropriate level. At this second signal, the cloths are removed and the operator begins the dermabrasion. Most of the time, the operator starts abrading at the periphery of the frozen area and moves toward its center. He abrades until he perceives the beginning of thawing of the tissue, since at that time there is an increased risk of gouging or running of the tip over the skin. When a given segment is completely abraded, the team then moves on to the next segment as indicated by the moving of the cloths, the previous painting with gentian violet, or an indication by the physician as to where he wants to abrade next. If the areas are indicated by the movement of cloths or towels, it is important to allow some overlap of the abrasion so that there is no gap between segments. This procedure continues under the direction of the operator until all of the areas have been completed. It is extremely important to protect the patient's eyes, nose, lips, and ears from the spraying. Some physicians prefer to do this by taping eye pads in place, placing petrolatum over the palpebral fissures or taping lead eye shields in place. Others, such as ourselves, try to keep it simple and cover the eyes with a cloth during freezing and then remove it when the abrasion starts.

Two freezing philosophies exist. The first is to spray on the cryogen with the skin in its normal state and under no tension. This way, the defects are frozen in place, and the operator dermabrades to the desired level of those defects. The opposite philosophy is to stretch the skin taut before spraying, realizing that the defects are frozen in an unnatural form and that the dermabrasion will take place over defects that are somewhat distorted.

In actuality, it seems that operators with either philosophy achieve good results. It is more a matter of paying careful attention to each spot that is dermabraded and watching the levels of the skin and at the base of the scar to be sure that the abrasion is carried to an appropriate depth. It matters little whether the defect was stretched before freezing, assuming that the operator is knowledgeable in the particular technique being used. The important factor is how deep the wound is carried and how well the scars are beveled to the surrounding skin.

WIRE BRUSH TECHNIQUE

Kurtin wire brushes are manufactured with a 17.0-mm diameter and four different widths: 3.0 mm, 6.0 mm, 9.0 mm, and 12.0 mm. The thickness of the stainless steel wire is regular (0.003 inch), coarse (0.004 inch), or fine (0.0025 inch). The most commonly used is the regular sized stainless steel wire (0.003 inch) on a medium (6.0-mm) brush.

All of the standard techniques described above for dermabrasion apply to the use of dermabrasion with the wire brush, except however, when using a wire brush, the skin *must* be frozen board hard. The wire brush never should be applied to tissue that is not board hard or that is beginning to thaw. Wire brushes applied to nonfrozen tissue will gouge out deep chunks of tissue, which can result in hypertrophic or atrophic scarring. Literally, lips and eyelids have been torn, and deep gouges on the cheeks and nose have been made when the hard freeze rule was not followed carefully.

Once the area is frozen and the towels or cloths are taken away, the operator begins to dermabrade the frozen surface, starting with the periphery, which will thaw the fastest, and moves toward the center. The best stroke for the beginner using a wire brush is to pull the dermabrasion handle lightly toward himself in short strokes (approximately 1.0 to 2.0 cm long). The handle always should be drawn across the skin at right angles to the plane of rotation. It never should be drawn across the skin in the same plane as the plane of rotation, since this more likely will result in a deep groove or gouge. This rule cannot be overstressed, particularly with the wire brush. Similarly, the beginning operator should not use a stroke in which he pushes the dermabrasion handle away from himself, since there is a natural tendency when pushing the brush away to angle the tip down into the skin, which easily can result in deeper and deeper abrasion. The experienced dermabrader may feel comfortable moving the brush in back-and-forth directions, but must pay careful attention to obtaining an equal depth of abrasion throughout. The unskilled dermabrader using a back-and-forth motion easily can leave a grooved look. Some dermabraders plane between the grooves whereas others redo the surface lightly at right angles to the first direction so that they avoid this effect. Still others use a circular motion of short, continuous circles to avoid any grooved appearance. To practice these various techniques, we strongly urge the use of the grapefruit laboratory device or a fresh pig's foot, frozen with cryogen. With practice and experience, it does not matter which technique is used, back and forth or circular. However, the warning cannot be too strong to obtain training before performing the technique on humans to avoid some of the disastrous mistakes of the past.

When dermabrading the upper part of the chin and the lower lip, it is helpful to have the patient place the tongue between the lower lip and teeth to produce a flatter surface. The nose can be dermabraded with the wire brush if the dermabrader is experienced. However, other end-pieces described below generally are much easier for the nasal and lip areas.

In the past, eyelids have been dermabraded, but we certainly do not recommend that anyone attempt to dermabrade the eyelids unless he truly is an expert. We have dermabraded on the eyelids with a fraise but always do so with worry and tension.

In doing wire brush dermabrasion, there is a danger in the middle of the jaw. It is believed that the facial artery crossing the mandible represents the equivalent of a hot pipe in a frozen mass. Since this area is a most common site for hypertrophic scarring after dermabrasion, some people believe that the blood in this large vessel defrosts part of the field and, therefore, this relatively softer portion of the frozen field is gouged out easily by the wire brush. Others believe that this area simply has thinner skin and is more easily dermabraded too deeply and that the causes of scarring have nothing to do with the vessel. Still others believe that the sharp curve over the jawbone itself is not adequately compensated for by the abrader and, again, the dermabrasion is carried too deeply. Pulling the jaw skin superiorly so a flat surface is abraded may reduce scarring.

While planning around orifices it is important that direction of rotation of the tip be toward the orifice. Therefore, the dermabrader may have to stand on the opposite side of the table when planing the skin of the lower lip or the upper lip or to have equipment that will rotate in both directions. The theory is that the abrading tip rotating toward the orifice essentially pushes the lip away rather than grabbing it and tearing it. The operator must be constantly aware of the direction of the rotating tip.

There always should be appropriate protection for the patient's eyes. Some dermabraders use eye shields cut out of lead. If a wire brush were to run toward the eyes, it would quickly bounce off this type of shield. Other operators use goggles similar to those used for swimming or for protection from ultraviolet radiation. We believe that to use a high-speed, whirling wire brush or any dermabrasion equipment around the eyes, the operator should be sufficiently skilled to prevent such problems. We are much more comfortable with simply holding a towel near the eyes when we are spraying and covering the closed eyes with a hand when we actually are abrading.

When using the wire brush, the handle of the instrument must be grasped more firmly than other devices, since this tip has the greatest tendency to run.

If there is any untoward event, it is good training for the dermabrader to learn to quickly take his foot off the foot pedal and simultaneously raise the dermabrading tip above his head. Patients who are startled sometimes bolt upright and can move right into the whirling tip. If the operator already has raised the equipment away from the patient and stopped the machine, there is less likelihood of damage.

The depth of dermabrasion with the wire brush is judged by the cutting action on the collagen. The stages described above for the grapefruit model pertain to diamond fraise dermabrasion. Dermabrasion with a wire brush is continued until the collagen frays. This is appreciated as linear separations within the frozen mass of the collagen compared with the smooth, even removal of tissue from the uppermost dermis with the diamond fraises. The fraying action of the wire brush does not usually permit one to see sebaceous glands as clearly as with other tips. Therefore, the abrasion continues down until the fraying of collagen is observed.[5]

Immediately following dermabrasion, a variety of hemostatic agents has been used. Topical thrombin soaks have been applied. These provide a smooth surface with minimal oozing when the patient leaves. However, this is costly and time-consuming. Collagen derivatives, such as Avitene sprinkled on the surface, provide essentially instantaneous coagulation and a dry surface. However, costs to cover a whole face are high. Hydrogen peroxide is used by some plastic surgeons who believe that it provides faster hemostasis. We are sure that styptic materials have been used. But we find none of these to be necessary. Washing the area of dermabrasion with Hibiclens soap postoperatively and applying an antibiotic ointment, Telfa, gauze, and a clean wrap dressing are all that is required. The antibiotic ointment could be deleted and Adaptic substituted for the Telfa. What is important is to use sound wound care and allow the dermabraded area to heal. The dressings are removed the following morning, although they can be left on for two days. Most patients find that the dressings become soaked with serum, so removing them adds a measure of comfort. If open healing is chosen, the patient may want to keep a towel around the neck for the first 24 to 48 hours to catch the oozing serum.

Healing after wire brush dermabrasion should take a minimum of seven to ten days, using the open healing method. If plastic dressings are applied, such as Op-Site, epithelization can occur sooner than seven days. It is important to appreciate that when pictures of full reepithelization in five days using an open method of healing are shown at lectures, real dermabrasion has not been performed, only superficial removal of a little tissue. Epidermabrasion is all that has been accomplished.

DIAMOND FRAISE TECHNIQUE

The most popular fraise is either the rough fraise from the regular-rough classification or the regular fraise from the fine-regular classification. The less-coarse diamond bits seem to offer no advantages but do have the disadvantage of removing tissue much more slowly. It is not uncommon to hear wire brush dermabraders criticize diamond fraise dermabraders, since they believe that it is nearly impossible to obtain a deep enough abrasion with the diamond fraise. This problem can easily be settled in every individual's mind by using the two instruments on a fresh pig's foot that has been frozen firmly with Freon spray.

The diamond fraise is quite able to abrade as deeply as one could want. It is true that the brush will cut faster, but the same depths can be obtained with little difficulty with a good freeze and a diamond fraise.

The fraise wheels come in diameters of 10.0 mm, 13.0 mm, 15.0 mm, and 17.0 mm, with widths of 2.5 mm, 4.0 mm, 6.0 mm, 8.0 mm, and 10.0 mm (Fig 4–13). Smaller specialized tips that are pear-shaped or bullet-shaped also are available. We are happiest with the standard fraises, which are not extremely wide. In our opinion, the very wide end-pieces do not provide the desired depth of cutting. They also do not allow the flexibility of rotating up on the edge of the fraise so that small areas can be abraded more deeply as needed. In our hands, we believe that the best results are obtained using the rough diamond fraise that is 4.0 mm wide and 17.0 mm in diameter. We believe that this is common among other dermatologists.

It would be helpful for each dermabrader to try the various types of end tips in a laboratory on pigs' feet or grapefruit. Then try several on patients and select the type or types that complement your own skills. Some physicians prefer the large, flat-surface wheels because they cover a wider area and there is less chance of grooving. However, with experience, most physicians find that the narrower end tips give them more latitude to abrade around and into various scars and defects while at the same time they have no difficulty performing a smooth abrasion. Holding the hand engine with the hand under the handle, it often is difficult to place the large, flat wheel perfectly flat to the skin. This is another reason some physicians prefer the use of a narrower end piece.

We almost always use the cone-shaped (bullet) or pear-shaped tips for part of a dermabrasion. They allow excellent maneuverability across the nasal ala and glabella, and we use them either as the first or last step of a full-face dermabrasion to abrade around individual scars and in pits. These small fraises can be used in a circular fashion; they have almost no tendency to run or gouge. The operator can hold the Bell hand engine like a pencil and "erase" small scars. For spot dermabrasions, this instrument and end-piece are superb.

The same basic motions as described for the brush are recommended for the fraise. Since the fraise cuts less deeply, the number of actual strokes will be increased. The most common stroke is a single stroke pulled toward the operator. However, as experience is gained, circular or back-and-forth motions per-

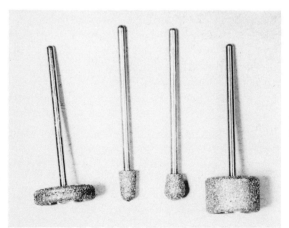

Fig 4–13.—Diamond fraises: *left*, round, usual type used; *second left*, bullet fraise; *third left*, pear fraise; *right*, wide, flat edge fraise.

pendicular to the diameter of the fraise are quite acceptable and speed the procedure greatly.

SERRATED WHEEL TECHNIQUE

Since these stainless steel wheels have sharp tips arranged in rows (Fig 4–14), they can catch on soft, loose skin and run just as wire brushes or sometimes even fraises. However, the tendency is far less and the cutting efficiency is quite similar to that of the brush. Although it is the least commonly used tip, the serrated wheel seems to represent the best features of both the fraise and the brush and theoretically would be the best instrument to use. Deep dermabrasion can be accomplished with little hand pressure, and light dermabrasion also is possible in the hands of an experienced operator. The same motions, indications, and contraindications as described for the wire brush

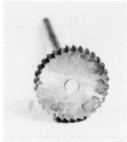

Fig 4–14.—Serrated wheel showing stainless steel teeth.

must be observed with the serrated wheels. One of us (T. A. T.), who has done a number of dermabrasions with all three methods, finds the serrated wheel the most comfortable for doing deep abrasions where there are many hard, elevated scars and the diamond fraise best for more superficial dermabrasions.

HIGH-SPEED DERMABRASION

The very high-speed machine, e.g., the Schreuss* (Derma III) machine mentioned above, utilizes diamond fraises and serrated wheels specially angled for this equipment. Because of the super-high speed at 60,000 rpm, cutting is accomplished more cleanly, and deeper dermabrasions can be obtained faster than with the other equipment described above. The total dermabrasion time can be reduced. The same short-stroke method directed toward the operator is used by beginners, the back-and-forth stroke or circular motion by the experts. The claim of individuals who use this machine is that it cuts deeper and quicker. No freezing is necessary, only three- or four-point traction, because the speed and torque provided by the high-speed machines do not allow the diamond chips to get caught in soft tissue, but cut the tissue cleanly away. In addition, since the tissue is cut faster and more cleanly, the edges of blood vessels in the skin are cut more evenly, and some thermal coagulation may occur at a microscopic level. This theoretically allows the body to seal the ends

---

*A. Schumann Precision Manufacturer, Concord, Mass.

of the vessels more quickly, resulting in less bleeding.[7] Using these high-speed machines, dermabrasion usually is done with the aid of general anesthesia. The opinion of those who have observed is that the dermabrasion is rapid and effective. Only the specific fraises recommended by the manufacturer should be used in the Schreus machine. Fraises of less-strong steel that are made for 30,000 rpm may show metal fatigue and result in the diamond wheel snapping off or bending and gouging. Using only recommended parts with the high-speed machines cannot be emphasized too strongly.

The credit for introducing these high-speed machines into the United States goes to Robert Stolar of Washington, D.C. He has more than a decade of experience with them and has helped to bring the machines to their present state of usefulness.[6]

Although we see benefit in the very high-speed machines, the cost of such equipment is five to seven times the cost of standard dermabrasion machines, making us recommend the standard machines for the beginner or the physician doing a low volume of dermabrasion. For someone doing a high volume of dermabrasion, it may be more practical to use the high-speed equipment, particularly if two or three dermabrasions can be done in one morning.

GENERAL PROCEDURE

We believe that, whenever possible, a full-face dermabrasion should be done. If scars exist in all cosmetic areas, it is easy to decide to do the full face. However, if parts of the face do not have scars, such as the nose, upper lip, forehead, or other cosmetic segments, a deeper dermabrasion can be done on the affected cosmetic units, with some contouring and light dermabrasion on the other areas. Some cosmetic surgeons combine the use of dermabrasion and a trichloroacetic acid or phenol peel. The belief is that in those areas that do not require dermabrasion, the peeling will help freshen the appearance of the skin, match the skin during healing (both areas will be wounded), and treat some of the actinic damage in the nonscarred areas because the dermabrasion itself will do that in the other areas.

However, one must warn the patient of the risks of both procedures. There always is the possibility that the peeling will lead to a different healing time with prolonged erythema. There definitely can be pigmentary changes from both techniques. We have had the misfortune of having several patients' skin become much lighter with dermabrasion and much darker with peeling. In one patient, when we combined the two during the same procedure, we ended up with an extremely unhappy patient because of the marked differences in the pigment over various cosmetic units. We finally had to do a dermabrasion over the entire face many months later—a long year and a half, for the patient, from the time of the initial treatment until the complete dermabrasion.

Except for patients with fair skin, we do not often recommend localized dermabrasions. It seems as though it should be easy to dermabrade small sections of the skin where there are just a few small scars. The problem is that there is a texture change and the risk of pigmentary change. The patient will have difficulty covering these changes with makeup, or if the patient does not use makeup, the spotted areas often show. We have many patients on whom we have successfully done localized dermabrasion, but it always is with trepidation that we undertake this task.

The main exception to our rule is small linear surgical scars, less than 2.0 cm long, or individual acne scars where the dermabraded area is approximately 1.0 cm in diameter. These spots usually assume normal color because of melanocyte migration from both the dermabraded follicles and the surrounding epidermis. Even if small areas of color change should develop, the trade-off of improving the scar appearance may be worthwhile, since most complexions are not a single even shade. Again, only 1.0- or 2.0-cm "test scars" should be treated initially to test that patient's response to spot dermabrasion.

POSTOPERATIVE CARE

There are innumerable recommended methods for postoperative care; some of them even seem contradictory. We keep telling ourselves that we make the wound, and the body heals the skin. It is our obligation only to assist in the healing, since the speed of healing has nothing to do with the final cosmetic outcome. We in no way want to impede this natural process.

We send patients home with antibacterial ointment, Telfa, and gauze (Fig 4–15). Then the simplest postoperative approach is to ask the patient to apply the antibiotic ointment two or three times a day. Some physicians recommend plain petrolatum and some recommend Crisco. The Crisco is kept in the refrigerator so that when it is applied it is cool and feels soothing. We have seen surface contamination with *Pseudomonas,* and so recommend ointment containing polymyxin or gentamicin. The petrolatum base of the antibiotic ointment keeps the crust soft and flexible, which prevents cracking with facial movement.

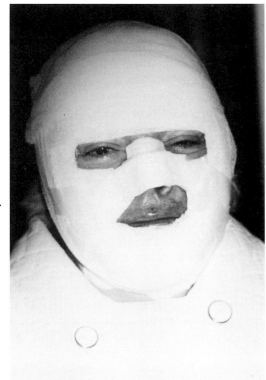

Fig 4–15.—Usual bandage immediately postdermabrasion.

We ask our patients to wash the face starting the second day—first only lightly, just splashing on water, followed by applying the ointment. By the third or fourth day, they are washing the face with mild soap and water and following with the antibiotic ointment.

There is a completely opposite school of postoperative dermabrasion care. Some physicians apply materials starting on the first postoperative day that will form a quick, thick crust. The famous thymol iodide powder has been a standby. We already have expressed that we do not believe this makes any difference. It is just one more medication and one more instruction to the patient that we believe is not of any benefit.

More recently, an emulsified petrolatum product, Hyperemollient, has been used. It is easier to put on than plain petrolatum, is nonirritating, speeds healing in laboratory tests, and is well liked by patients. Comparisons of dermabraded sites treated with Hyperemollient vs. Crisco, vegetable oils, mineral oil, and commercial dry-skin products showed that the Hyperemollient-treated sites always healed faster.*

Another new approach is the use of Debrisan Beads. These are small, synthetic dextran beads that make a hydroscopic layer. When placed on a moist wound, water is drawn along microscopic tunnels that form among the beads. Bacteria actually are drawn off the surface of the wound into the moist gel-like mask that is formed. Physicians using Debrisan Beads like them a great deal. The disadvantages are: they are slippery when dropped on the floor; messy to use; and must be discontinued when the wound changes from wet to dry, since they can irritate and slow the healing in dry wounds. Debrisan is costly, and, we believe, unnecessary. There is no doubt that this material removes moisture and bacteria from the wound, but that is of no real necessity postdermabrasion.

Op-Site and Biobrane are new surgical dressings that provide some special benefits. The biggest benefit is that the postoperative burning pain is reduced or completely eliminated. Op-Site is a polyurethane material with an adhesive that will stick to stratum corneum but not to wet wounds. When using this, it is necessary to have a nonabraded section of skin around the hairline and in the preauricular area so that the Op-Site can stick. On the other hand, Biobrane will stick to moist wounds and can be placed over the completely dermabraded face. Op-Site is much less expensive than Biobrane at the time of the writing of this book.

Manufacturers believe that these materials will not only increase comfort to the patient but will reduce wound infection and increase the speed of healing. The only problem we have had with these materials is that in some patients the number of milia increased when dressings were on for more than one week. In one patient there were more milia than we have ever seen. There is no reason why Op-Site cannot be used for two to three days and then replaced with the ointment-covered, open treatment. This will give the patient the benefit of reduced pain the first few days, followed by more comfortable open scabbing in the later phase of healing. Using Op-Site in this way has not produced increased numbers of milia.

Again, we are faced with the same dilemma, since none of these methods

---

*Tests reported by Ivy Laboratories, Philadelphia.

really improves the cosmetic effect of dermabrasion and all of them add cost and hassle for the patient. Thus, we prefer our open ointment postoperative care. In this case, we see no reason why the simplest procedure is not the best.

POSTOPERATIVE FOLLOW-UP

Because they appear so unsightly, it is helpful for patients to have everything at hand when they leave the office so that they will have everything they need in their homes during the early phases of healing. We find that written instructions, along with oral ones, are helpful. We send the written instructions to the patients before the dermabrasion so that they can ask questions before they have any preoperative medication and before they become involved in the anxiety of the day and either forget to question or forget the answers.

We also give the patient postoperative "CARE packages." These include Tylenol with codeine, 30 mg, from our own office supply (it is much easier to give the patients this medication than to give them a prescription that they often will not fill immediately and then have to call that night because of the pain and discomfort), Hyperemollient and/or an antibiotic ointment, sterile Telfa pads, 3 × 3 cotton gauze squares, extra Kling bandages, and some adhesive tape. All of this gives the patient the option of putting on a fresh bandage either later that day or the next day. The fresh bandage, which is drier, makes them much more comfortable, makes them look better, and gives them a feeling of confidence. Quite frankly, providing such a package shows the patient that the physician cares and is not going to be "cheap" about a few supplies that could make the patient much more comfortable.

We prefer to see the patients 2 or 3 days after dermabrasion and again at 7 to 14 days. They can come to the office with a veil or scarf over the head and prearrange entry through the back door. Now that we are having the patients use Hyperemollient and an antibiotic ointment and keep the scabs as minimized as possible, they really do not always look that bad a week to 10 days after surgery. With many patients, we can answer questions over the telephone and thus have contact with them during the first postoperative days without their needing to come to the office.

As expected, if we can describe to the patients what will happen to them and then those events happen, their confidence in us increases and their own anxiety about the results diminishes. We are careful to tell the patients several times to expect a massively swollen face for the first few days after surgery. We also describe and show pictures of typical scabbing so that they will realize that it is normal. It is important to tell them that their eyes often will swell shut and that there may be some swelling in the neck and the submandibular area. Some patients find it much more comfortable to sleep with the head on two pillows, which allows gravity to draw the fluid away from the face and eyes. On the other hand, if patients find that they cannot sleep comfortably in that position, a good night's rest in the most natural position probably is better for them, even though they might have more of a problem with edema.

Some physicians routinely give corticosteroids following dermabrasion. We have not been convinced that this makes a significant difference in postoperative edema. As with many other substances, the users are absolutely convinced that it is helpful, but without the support of a controlled study; our negative belief is equally passionate, also without a controlled study.

The patient is instructed to remove the dressing the morning after the dermabrasion, clean up any ooze and exudate around the abrasion, and lightly pat to clean the dermabraded area. Then the Hyperemollient or antibiotic ointment is applied three to four times a day. Gradually, the patient will use more warm, soapy water to cleanse the face throughout the day, followed by an application of the ointment. We encourage the patient to keep the crusts soft and pliable and tell him that he may start to remove the crusts gently when they seem to come off easily.

Some physicians instruct patients not to move the face any more than necessary. We suspect that this may have some slight advantage for people with very mobile facial expressions. On the other hand, the edema immobilizes the face somewhat and probably is just as effective in restricting facial movements.

We tell patients that the crusts will come off in ten to 14 days and that, after that, the face will be extremely bright pink or red. They can start applying cover makeup as soon as the scabs are off, and it may require some professional makeup advice on how to completely cover the bright pink skin for the first month or so after dermabrasion. We encourage patients to wait a minimum of two weeks before returning to activities that expose them to the public. Naturally, working patients try to schedule the procedure on a Friday and return to work about ten days later. This leaves a marginal, recovery period, though, and we do not recommend it.

All patients are carefully and repeatedly instructed about avoiding direct or strong sunlight for three to six months. Although dermabrasion is accomplished without problems in sunny areas such as Hawaii if appropriate sunscreens and cover makeup are used, in the temperate climates with notable changes in seasons it is helpful to perform dermabrasion in the late fall through the early spring so that avoidance of strong sun is easier. Premature suntanning increases the incidence of hyperpigmentation. Although hyperpigmentation almost always is temporary, it is unsightly, bothersome, and requires some sort of cover-up. If it can be avoided by staying out of strong sunlight, that certainly is the better approach. It is important that patients understand the problems with reflective light as well as direct light. Brief exposure to sunlight reflected from snow or water presents a large dose of ultraviolet light to the surface of the skin.

COMPLICATIONS OF DERMABRASION

Scarring as the result of excessive freezing is most likely a complication of dermabrasion, but it is difficult to prove in the clinical situation. This possibility is discussed in meetings, and several very experienced dermabraders believe that it is possible. On the other hand, studies on both humans and animals separate the wound of freezing from the wound of dermabrasion. In guinea pigs the freeze adds to the depth of the dermabrasion injury if it lasts longer than 20 seconds and is repeated after thawing (unpublished guinea pig study by S. J. S.). In humans the lack of wounding from light freezing has been shown, but a study to demonstrate whether dermabrasion and the freeze injury are additive has not been published. There has been one oral report at a meeting that multiple hard freezes with Freon-12 have induced scarring in a thin skin area in an experimental situation. Theoretically, if part of the epidermis and upper dermis had been dermabraded off and another freeze applied to the same area, this second freezing possibly would extend the wound deep enough into the subcutaneous tissue to increase the scarring potential. In summary, we believe that it is possible to obtain scarring from deep freezing in dermabrasion. However, from our experience, we believe that this is probably very unlikely and do refreeze the same area when necessary.

Metal fatigue of the shaft of the dermabrading tip is a real and serious danger. The shaft may suddenly bend and there is a risk of gouging out tissue, or the tip may break off and become a dangerous airborne missile. We are aware of both of these events having happened during dermabrasion.

There are two ways to help prevent this complication. One is to inspect the dermabrading tip carefully and test it before starting each procedure. The tip should be placed in the machine and turned to its highest revolution setting and the rotating end carefully examined to be sure that it is not wobbling or shaking. It also should become standard procedure to discard any tips that are worn either at their abrading end or along the metal shaft.

Scarring probably is the most important complication of dermabrasion. These scars are almost always hypertrophic, but we have seen true keloid formation (fortunately, not on our own patients). It is difficult to estimate the incidence of hypertrophic scarring. There is no doubt that the incidence is greater on the jawline, frequently midway between the chin and the angle of the jaw, and on the upper one-half of the upper lip (Fig 4–16).

There are several theories as to why the skin on the jawline is more susceptible to scarring. One is the "hot pipe" theory which applied to wire brush dermabraders because a less frozen area was easily gouged out. However, we

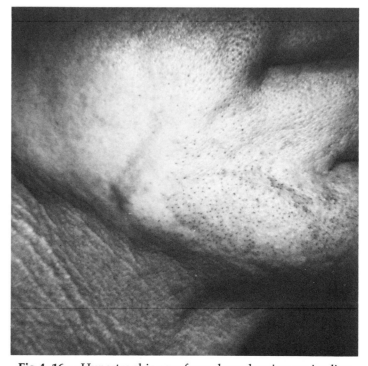

Fig 4–16.—Hypertrophic scar from dermabrasion on jawline.

also find that the jawline is the area most often scarred in working with diamond fraises. For the diamond fraise dermabrader, if the skin is less frozen, the wound would be more shallow. Thus, we are not convinced that the facial artery ''hot pipe'' theory is valid.

Another possibility is that the skin is thinner, with less subcutaneous fat, as it crosses over the jawline. This could account for an unsuspected deeper wound at this area.

Yet another theory is that the skin is more movable over the jawline and exposed to the stresses of movement as the patient talks and masticates. Clearly, movement of skin does contribute to increased scar formation if there is a deeper wound or more tension across the wound.

Treatment for scars is injection with triamcinolone acetonide, starting at 5–10 mg/ml and increasing to 20 mg/ml. Only rarely do we find the need for 40 mg/ml. Because there is a potential of build-up of steroid crystals in the tissue, we limit injections to every four to six weeks. In our experience we have had excellent results with this treatment in all cases but one. We were consulted on a keloid problem (in a Mexican-American who underwent dermabrasion in Mexico). After several years of repeated injections, the scars flattened enough so that the patient could cover them satisfactorily with makeup.

We have seen the pictures and heard the discussions by John Yarborough of New Orleans. Yarborough has a long experience with dermabrasion and advises that one should inspect the dermabraded area at one week and two weeks after crusts are off. If there are any focal areas of increased redness, he immediately applies Cordran tape. The tape is worn for eight hours a day until the site is no longer more erythematous than the surrounding skin. Although Yarborough has not done a paired comparison for this preventive treatment suggestion, his clinical observation is that he has prevented or treated hypertrophic scarring as it developed.

The second most serious complication is altered pigmentation, hypopigmentation being the more common after dermabrasion (Fig 4–17). It is not surprising that dermabrasion leads to hypopigmentation, since the technique not only removes the melanocytes in the basement membrane, but also removes many of the melanocytes that are in the external root sheath. Also, melanocytes are sensitive to freezing and might be destroyed with even a very superficial dermabrasion if there was enough freezing.

Among dermatologists who were dermabrading in the 1960s and 1970s, it was more common to obtain a characteristic pasty-white skin postdermabrasion. This was believed to be related to the deeper freezes and to deep dermabrasions by the wire brush. More recently, dermabrasion seems to be done to a more moderate depth, since it gives an equally good cosmetic result. Thus, the characteristic pasty-white look is not seen as often.

The regional dermabrasion or the dermabrasion of a portion of one cosmetic unit creates the biggest problem for the patient if there are pigmentary changes. The texture difference of the skin after dermabrasion, particularly if the patient has a great deal of actinic damage, is also more noticeable with regional or a portion of a cosmetic unit dermabrasion. These smaller procedures probably should be limited to those individuals who have a very fair complexion, minimal sun damage, or who routinely wear makeup.

Hyperpigmentation problems are seen in two forms. The first is the hyperpigmented line at the boundary between the nondermabraded and derma-

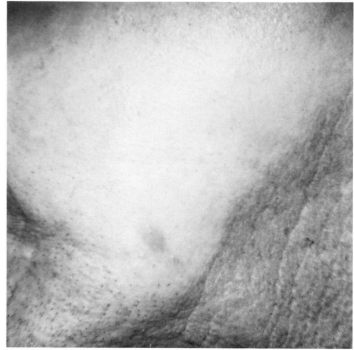

Fig 4–17.—Hypopigmentation following dermabrasion.

braded skin. The theory is that at the edge of the dermabraded area, the skin was only partially frozen and the dermabrasion was feathered, leading to a sublethal injury to the melanocytes. This sublethal injury then results in hyperpigmentation rather than depigmentation. Support for this theory is that those physicians who use no freezing for dermabrasion rarely see this line, as do physicians who dermabrade with the fraise just beyond the frozen edge.

The second form of hyperpigmentation is the spotted type or the pinto pony look. This is most likely postinflammatory hyperpigmentation and is seen more commonly in patients with moderately dark complexions, such as Micronesians, Mediterraneans, or light blacks. This same hyperpigmentation is seen in the patient who receives too much solar radiation during the first three months postdermabrasion.

Fortunately, most of the postinflammatory hyperpigmentation fades over the first six months, although we have seen it take up to two years in some patients. One of the reasons to do a test spot is to demonstrate each patient's likelihood of forming hyperpigmentation. Patients also find out how long it will take that hyperpigmentation to fade, which gives them a better realization of the total amount of time involved in the procedure. Several times patients have had deeply hyperpigmented test spots, which we both were very happy to see because it saved us a great deal of anguish later.

Milia are probably the commonest side effect of dermabrasions; a few milia can be expected in almost every patient. If left alone for several months, all milia spontaneously will disappear. However, patients usually prefer to have them treated (Fig 4–18). They can be incised with a #11 blade or Hagadorn needle. Our method is lightly to touch the top of the milia with a hot cautery (direct current) with the heat set very low. This produces a tiny burn on the top of the milia, which results in drainage and leaves no residual mark. We

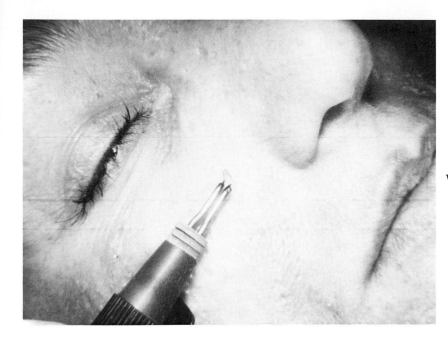

Fig 4–18.—Milia being treated with hot cautery.

also have successfully applied chemical cauterants such as phenol or 50% trichloroacetic acid, but the hot cautery is the fastest, the most efficient, and the easiest to use.

A variety of other side effects occasionally is seen. Grooving of the skin is a most unpleasant side effect and probably is directly related to the skill of the dermabrader. If long strokes were used and not later abraded over with circular or perpendicular strokes, there might be a long groove in the skin after complete healing. There is no treatment for this except to redermabrade. Grooving is more likely if the freeze was hard and the dermabrasion was deep.

Sometimes, if the dermabrasion was carried to unequal depths, there is a patchy look to the skin. Fortunately, this tends to even out after four to six months.

Sometimes purpura develops beneath the new epidermis; usually this is noticed within the first month. We presume that this is due to a shearing force applied to the new epidermis resulting in epidermal separation and tearing of the new vessels. Fortunately, this, too, heals spontaneously.

Acne may become better or worse following dermabrasion. Most of the time, people with active acne notice an increase in the acne activity during the first few months postdermabrasion. They should continue their regular acne treatments as much as possible. Other patients who have comedonal acne usually notice a clearing of a certain percent of those closed comedones.

Lupus erythematosus lesions have been activated by dermabrasion, but this is uncommon. We wait for the discoid lesions to be in remission for at least one year before considering dermabrasion.

True infection rarely is seen and has readily responded to erythromycin or semisynthetic penicillin with no permanent untoward effects on the outcome of the abrasion. Occasionally, a green surface growth from *Pseudomonas* is seen. This is not true infection and responds to topical polymyxin or topical gentamicin.

Almost all of the side effects of dermabrasion are treatable. It is far better to prevent side effects by proper use and care of equipment, always appreciating the magnitude of a dermabrasion procedure, having detailed information on all aspects of the specific procedure, obtaining laboratory practice, attendance at specialized dermabrasion courses such as those given by the American Society for Dermatologic Surgery, and spending sufficient time at the side of someone truly knowledgeable in the specific technique of dermabrasion you plan to do. Shortcuts in these steps invite unnecessary, preventable side effects.

REFERENCES

1. Stegman S.J.: A comparative histologic study of the effects of three peeling agents and dermabrasion on normal and sun-damaged skin. *Aesth. Plast. Surg.* 1983 (in press).
2. Wilson J.W., Luikart R. II, Ayres S.W. III: Dichlorotetrafluoroethane for surgical planing. *Arch. Dermatol.* 71:523, 1955.
3. Wilson J.W., Ayres S.W. III, Luikart R. II: Mixtures of fluorinated hydrocarbons as refrigerant anesthetic. *Arch. Dermatol.* 74:310, 1956.
4. Ayres S., III, Wilson J.W., Luikart R. II: Dermal changes following abrasion. *Arch. Dermatol.* 79:553–568, 1959.
5. Burks J., Farber G.: *Dermabrasion and Chemical Peel: In the Treatment of Certain Cosmetic Defects and Diseases of the Skin.* Springfield, Ill., Charles C Thomas, Publisher, 1979.
6. Fulton J.E. Jr.: Dermabrasion by diamond fraises at 85,000 revolutions per minute. *J. Dermatol. Surg. Oncol.* 4:777–779, 1978.
7. Stolar R., Washington, D.C. Personal communication.
8. Abadir, D.M., Abadir A.R.: Dermabrasion under regional anesthesia without refrigeration of the skin. *J. Dermatal. Surg. Oncol.* 6:119–121, 1980.
9. Epstein E.: Dermabrasion, in Epstein E., Epstein E. Jr. (eds.): *Skin Surgery.* Springfield, Ill., Charles C Thomas, Publisher, 1982, pp. 593–611.
10. Rees T.D., Wood-Smith D.: *Cosmetic Facial Surgery.* Philadelphia, W.B. Saunders Co., 1973, pp. 213–231.
11. Rees T.D.: *Aesthetic Plastic Surgery.* Philadelphia, W.B. Saunders Co., 1980, pp. 749–769.

5 / Punch Grafts for Alopecia

THERE ARE FOUR major methods for the surgical management of male pattern alopecia: Orentreich punch grafts, Vallis strip grafts, scalp reduction, and flaps. Each of these methods is discussed in individual chapters.

ORENTREICH PUNCH GRAFT METHOD FOR MALE PATTERN ALOPECIA

The method popularized by Dr. Norman Orentreich in New York City was published in 1959 and is known as the Orentreich punch graft method.[1,2] For several years he had been studying causes of diseases, particularly diseases of the hair, by exchanging punch grafts among affected and unaffected areas with appropriate controls. He found that donor dominance existed in male pattern alopecia and evolved a theory that each individual hair has a genetic predisposition to be lost at a certain age or to be retained for life. In general there seemed to be two major groups of hairs on the scalp: the fringe hairs, which do not undergo miniaturization, and those on the top of the scalp, which, in patients who are programed for baldness, gradually miniaturize and finally stop growing. The difference in their biologic behavior is well demonstrated by the man who is totally bald on the crown but has thick fringe hair, compared with those patients who have the form of alopecia areata called ophiasis, in which all of the fringe hair is lost but the hair on the top of the scalp continues to grow.

It was in the late 1950s and early 1960s that Orentreich, and then Orentreich and Berger, undertook numerous trials entailing a variety of punch sizes, shapes, and cutting edges. From their studies and punch designs by Noel Robbins evolved modern hair transplantation.

PATIENT SELECTION

Patient selection is as important as the surgical skill needed to perform hair transplants. The patient should be a stable individual who understands what the technique will and will not accomplish. Patients should realize and accept that the hair never can be as thick as it once was and that hair transplants will not make them younger. They must appreciate that hair transplantation only redistributes hair from the back and sides over the top and front. They must be doing the procedure *for themselves*. If there is any suggestion that another person, such as a spouse or lover, wants them to have hair transplants, we suggest that they bring that party to the consultation. The patient should be warned of the statistical probability of all side effects and of negative features.

Patients who have been forewarned of the possible side effects and limitations can more readily maintain a good physician-patient relationship so that any undesirable effect can be corrected. Even after the most scrupulous screening, some patients will be dissatisfied, so it is wise to be certain that the screening process is thorough.

The best candidates, male or female, are those who understand that their transplantation will not make them younger and cannot restore their original hair, but may improve their appearance.

PREPARATION OF THE PATIENT

Taking a good general medical history is important, with special inquiry into bleeding or healing problems and diseases that affect the scalp. Laboratory work might consist of a CBC and urinalysis, bleeding and clotting time and an SMA-12 or SMA-23 blood screening test. Some physicians require hepatitis screening tests and will not accept patients whose results are positive.

Patients with normal laboratory test results still may bleed excessively. For this reason, we do not rely on laboratory tests alone and one of us prefers to do four to ten test plugs. Although the time lag sometimes is annoying to the patient, test plugs are the best means of predicting what problems might arise in doing large numbers of transplants, and the patient can judge these problems and aftercare from this small set. We tell patients that they can have large numbers of transplants done two weeks or more after the initial trial set. To the patient, this is not a significant delay, and it enables us to gather information and outline a smooth postoperative course.

Usually the patients wash their hair with their favorite shampoo the morning of or the night before hair transplants are done. Some physicians have the patient's hair washed in the office with an antibacterial cleanser immediately before hair transplantation to reduce the total amount of bacteria on the scalp and thereby reduce the possibility of infection. It now is appreciated that the

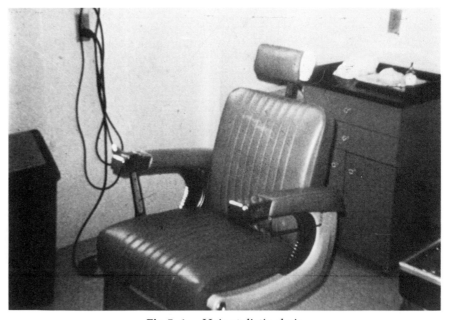

Fig 5–1.—Hair stylist's chair.

incidence of infection is low and readily handled. Simple washing at home is all that is required.

Transplants may be done with the patient in street clothes or in a surgical gown. The patient may lie flat or with the head slightly elevated on a regular surgical table, or may sit upright in a surgical or hair stylist's chair, as shown in Figure 5–1. We have found a hair stylist's chair best for our procedure. The chair can turn and be elevated or tilted, if necessary, to handle syncope. The physician sees the patients as they are in life, upright, and the psychologic distress of the operation lessens somewhat, since the patients are sitting upright, in street clothes, and know that they will be able to drive themselves home.

The hair on the posterior or sides of the scalp, the donor site, is lifted up, and an appropriately sized area is trimmed short with scissors or a barber's hair clipper. Small Metzenbaum scissors work well, and you may want one pair for this purpose only. The area must not be shaved, since the surgeon needs approximately 3.0–5.0 mm of hair length to ascertain the angles at which the hair emerges from the scalp. Hair spicules are removed from the donor area with a dry, surgical hand-washing brush, by application of tape that adheres to the loose spicules or by a vacuum machine.

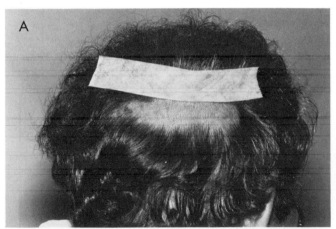

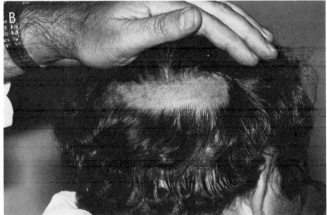

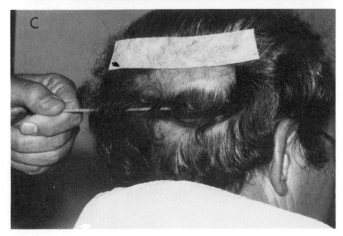

Fig 5–2.—**A**, hair taped up superior to donor area. **B**, rectangular donor area. **C**, double row donor area.

Hair superior to the donor site can be kept out of the operative field by hair clips, combs placed backward, or by Micropore or Dermicel tape (Fig 5–2,A). Some surgeons use a rectangular donor area as shown in Figure 5–2,B. Other surgeons alternate areas of trimmed hair wide enough to take two rows of plugs with areas of untrimmed hair, moving downward on the scalp (Fig 5–2,C). Surgeons who prefer the latter approach believe that hair coverage of the donor area in the immediate postoperative period is enhanced and is worth the added time and care needed to trim discrete areas. Do not plan donor areas with the long axis of the rectangle lying cephalocaudad, since the donor area will be seen for several months until the hair has grown long enough to hide it.

ANESTHESIA

Our first choice for local anesthesia is 1% lidocaine with 1:100,000 epinephrine. Up to 50 ml of the 1% concentration can be safely used before toxic levels are reached. Where the 50-ml limit may be approached because the whole top of the head must be anesthetized, 0.5% lidocaine is made by diluting the 1% lidocaine with epinephrine with saline for injection. Both concentrations seem to work well. A line or ring of anesthesia is injected into the subcutaneous tissue below the donor and recipient areas or around the whole scalp. The midline frontal area at the hairline often is difficult to anesthetize. Sometimes anesthesia can be achieved by injecting additional 1% lidocaine with epinephrine at the intradermal level. At other times, we find that reinjection of the same area with 1% mepivacaine (Carbocaine) will produce adequate anesthesia.

Some surgeons use 2% lidocaine in the frontal area or for all of the areas. We have not found any additional value to justify the increased total dosage of lidocaine, which increases the possibility of toxic reactions.

When using the power punch, swell the donor area with 10.0–30.0 ml of physiologic saline. This seems to result in less bleeding and less chance that the power punch will strike the skull. The saline injections may straighten the hair shafts further so that when plugs are cut, fewer roots are transected.

Sometimes we make the lidocaine-epinephrine mixture in our office. A 0.1-ml volume of 1:1,000 aqueous epinephrine per 10 ml of plain lidocaine will give a final epinephrine concentration of 1:100,000. Fresh solutions made this way seem to decrease the sting of injection. Factory-made lidocaine with epinephrine is titrated to a pH of 3.0–3.5 to maintain stability of the epinephrine molecule during storage. Plain lidocaine has a pH of 6.8 and, therefore, is closer to physiologic pH. Freshly made anesthetic should be used within 24–48 hours because the epinephrine molecule undergoes degradation and will not produce the hemostasis desired. We find it most convenient to add 0.2 ml of 1:1,000 aqueous epinephrine to a bottle containing 20 ml of plain lidocaine. That is a sufficient amount of local anesthetic for most patients. On using the whole bottle, we have an automatic reminder of the amount of anesthetic used. There may be some waste, since a fresh bottle is prepared for each hair transplant patient. If two or more sets of transplants are to be done the same day, the preparation of a 50-ml bottle of lidocaine may be more advantageous. Also, warming the solution to body temperature decreases its sting.

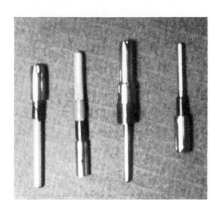

Fig 5–3.—Hair transplant punches. *Left,* Orentreich type with long linear grooves parallel to handle; *second left,* Resnik-Lewis punch with diamond cross-cut knurled handle; *third left,* Australian power punch; *right,* American power punch.

When taking donor plugs by the manual method, we use Orentreich punches with the handles modified with diamond crosscut grips, as described by Resnik and Lewis, with diameters of 1.5–6.0 mm (Fig 5–3). For most patients, a 4.5-mm diameter plug placed into a 4.0-mm or 4.25-mm recipient hole is our favorite combination. Larger donor diameters of 5.0–6.0 mm have produced reasonably good cosmetic results; however, the central portion of the plug did not grow in approximately 40% of the transplants. Although some patients like the "big bush" effect, the loss of hairs in the center of the plugs, along with additional bleeding and greater area of scar formation in the donor area, led us to prefer the 4.5-mm size. This size always is used when the hair in the donor area is thinner than average. The object is to include the maximum possible number of hairs per plug. For blending, creating more natural hairlines, or filling in on a patient whose hair is thinning only on the top, a 4.0-mm donor plug into a 3.5-mm recipient hole is our routine.

We use internal bevel punches as described by Hagerman and Wilson[3] (Fig 5–4,A). External bevel punches of the type commonly used in the United States produce peg-shaped or cone-shaped plugs, with the narrowest diameter at the level of the hair root. This results in fewer roots than shafts and, thus, fewer final hairs per graft (Fig 5–4,B). A punch is available in Australia with the outside and inside edges both beveled to a 20-degree angle (Fig 5–4,C). A 20-degree angle is known to hold the sharpest edge. The Australian punch produces plugs with greater numbers of hair roots. However, if you look at the punches on end, so that you are seeing the diameters of the cutting edges, the Australian punches labeled 4.5 mm have larger diameters than the American punches labeled 4.5 mm. Obviously, a larger-diameter punch will produce plugs with a larger diameter and more hairs. Whether this actual size discrepancy is due to different measurement techniques used in the United States and Australia is not clear. For example, it might be standard for one country labeling a punch 4.5 mm to be indicating external diameter whereas a 4.5-mm punch from the other country might indicate the internal diameter. Obviously, the one with a 4.5-mm internal diameter would produce larger plugs with more hairs.

Also, different manufacturers' drilling machines may vary slightly. Since punches are manufactured starting with a solid piece of stainless steel, slight differences in drilling pieces can produce different internal diameters. The study needed is not to compare punches from different manufacturers but to

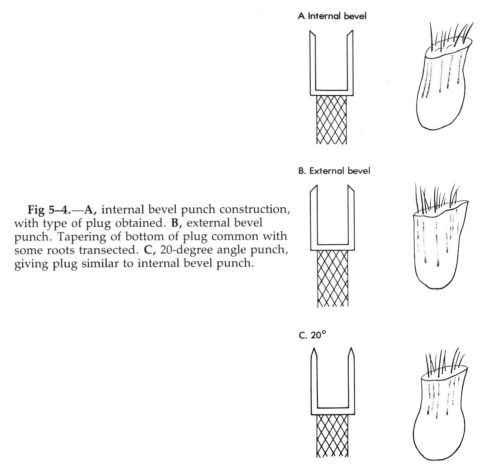

Fig 5–4.—**A,** internal bevel punch construction, with type of plug obtained. **B,** external bevel punch. Tapering of bottom of plug common with some roots transected. **C,** 20-degree angle punch, giving plug similar to internal bevel punch.

have one manufacturer make all the 4.5-mm punches. Some would then be ground on the edge to provide external bevels, others ground with internal bevels, and others with 20-degree angle bevels. Then a comparison of plugs taken with each type under the same conditions of saline bloating from the same donor area would settle the discussion as to which type is best. Until then, be sure to compare the cutting diameters of your punches as well as those of the "new punches" when someone says that the newer type is better. The newer type may be only slightly larger.

Rows of plugs are taken (Fig 5–5), starting with the lowest row and moving upward so that blood runs down, away from the donor row being worked on. Offsetting each row one-half space leaves hair immediately above a donor site, covering the scar. It also sets up an easy pattern for suturing two rows vertically or one or more rows horizontally with one running suture (Fig 5–6).

We routinely suture only those individual donor sites with active arterial or significant venous bleeding. Donor sites with bleeding that does not run out of the donor hole can be plugged with a rolled-up piece of Gelfoam sponge or left alone. If the patient cannot wear a head wrap, we close the donor area with a running suture of 3-0 white Mersilene. Braided sutures are more comfortable but require at least a 3-0 stength. A variation of the running suture, described by Dr. Harold Pierce, is shown in Figure 5–7. The skin bridges be-

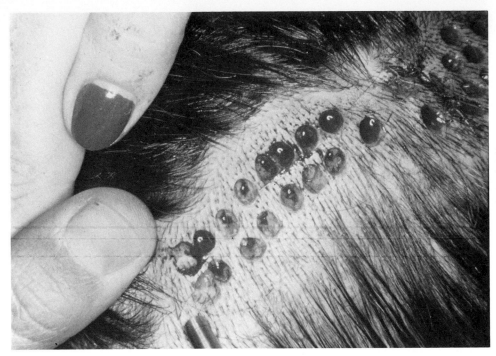

Fig 5–5.—Cutting plugs from donor area. Note, taking a lower-row plug before taking the next upper-row plug. (Gloves are worn now during this surgery.)

Fig 5–6.—*Left*, running suture to close single row of plugs. *Right*, running suture to close two donor holes with each loop of suture. →

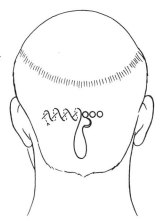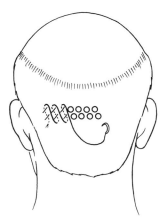

Fig 5–7.—Pierce suture closure. *Left*, donor holes showing proposed tiny incision lines to make one single wound. *Middle*, resultant wound after cutting into adjacent holes. *Right*, end scar line after suturing each inferior tip to superior concavity. ↓

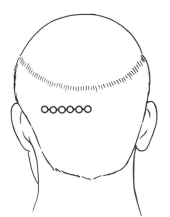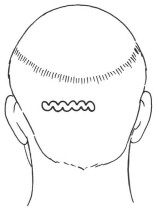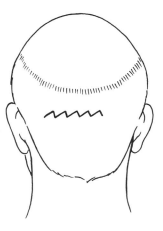

tween adjacent punches are cut and the holes sutured in a tongue-and-groove manner.

In the first few months postoperatively, the donor sites of patients who had suturing by regular methods always look better than sites that were not sutured; but after a year, the two are indistinguishable. However, the Pierce method shows a narrow line at a year and is preferred by many surgeons. A few surgeons suture active bleeding sites, use Gelfoam plugs in individual donor sites, and leave the other donor holes alone without even the use of a pressure head wrap. Others place the necessary sutures, then sprinkle fluffy Gelfoam powder over the entire donor area and cover with a head wrap. This forms a continuous soft layer, which usually will peel off in one piece on the following day. Other surgeons use Coban, a paper wrap that derives its elasticity from an overlapping and folding design. In our hands, Coban caused excessive pressure, leading to headaches in a number of patients. For us, the typical donor site dressing consists of white Telfa pads with an antibiotic ointment dotted on them (this has the additional advantage of helping the pads momentarily stick to the donor site), several layers of 3 × 3 mesh gauze in overlapping fashion, and a Kling bandage wrapped around the forehead and pulled firmly under the lambdoid ridge (Fig 5–8). We have not found it necessary to place the bandage beneath the chin, although this is sometimes recommended. Bandaging the recipient area is not necessary, but many patients believe that it is preferable for appearance' sake. We never use the bandage over the recipient area as a pressure wrap or to hold the plugs flatly in place; rather, it is used only for aesthetic purposes. Proper placement must be done at the time of insertion of plugs and checked before the final dressing. In the recipient area, the plug in place prevents bleeding except for an occasional arterial pumper, which requires a suture.

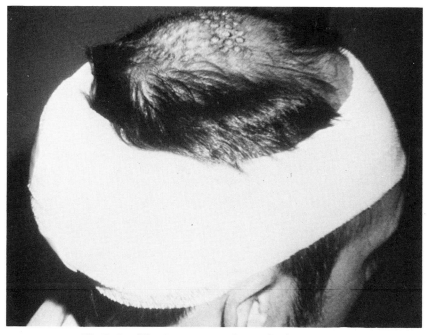

Fig 5–8.—Head wrap covering only donor area.

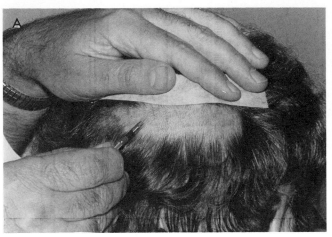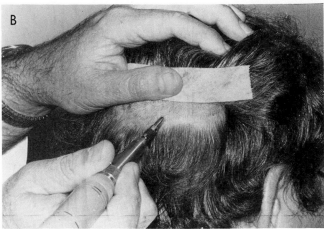

Fig 5–9.—**A,** cutting plugs with hand punch. Note that the angle of punch parallels angle of hair exiting from scalp. **B,** cutting plug with power punch. Note that the punch parallels hair shafts. (Gloves are worn now during this surgery.)

The donor plugs may be taken with either a hand punch (Fig 5–9,A) or a power punch (Fig 5–9,B). Equally good plugs with the same number of growing hairs can be obtained by either method, provided that punches are kept sharp. Power punch plugs may look thicker when sitting in the Petri dish, but studies by Unger[4] have shown that the same number of hairs grow from power or hand punches of equal diameters.

A variety of punch handles have been developed for hand punches. We prefer the original Orentreich type with the Resnik and Lewis grip variation (see Fig 5–3), in which a turning rather than a pushing action is used to obtain the plug. The original Orentreich punch had parallel longitudinal grooves, the Resnik and Lewis had a crosscut knurl, and the Stough has a wider and cone-shaped handle. Which to use is an individual preference.

The original description of cutting a plug was to aim perpendicular to the scalp, at least through the epidermis, and then lower the handle of the punch so that the barrel was parallel to the hairs. It is much better to have extremely sharp punches so that the initial contact of the scalp edge with the punch is in a plane parallel to the growth of the hairs.

Remove several of the first plugs taken to see that they are being cut parallel to the hairs and that there are no transected hair shafts at the periphery of the grafts. Inspection of the plugs should be done several times throughout the harvesting of these grafts. If transected hairs are found, correct the angle of approach. Shafts without roots will not grow hairs, and roots with the pilosebaceous channel cut away may not grow and may cause foreign-body reactions. Transecting roots is a common source of poor hair growth. Wearing a magnifying head visor helps visualize the direction of the hairs and improves the chances of obtaining excellent plugs. Simple half-frame 1.50 magnifying ''reading'' glasses purchased at the drugstore for approximately $10 also work well.

The Bell International hand engine, model 5B or 25D, is the most commonly used power device. Hold it as you would a pencil for the lightest and most accurate touch. As with a sharp hand punch, initial entry into the skin is par-

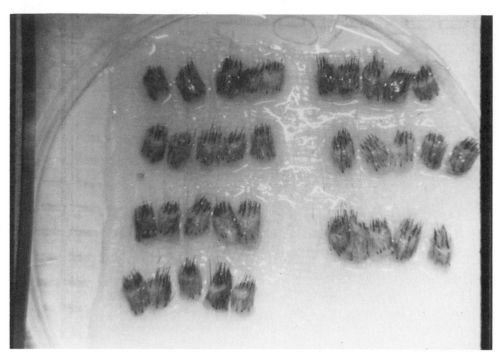

Fig 5–10.—Plugs in Petri dish in groups of five. Note evenness of width of plugs taken with internal bevel punch.

allel to the hair shafts (see Fig 5–9,B). Other dermabrasion machines and the Concept Company battery power unit can be used. These power units operate best with power punch handles that are machined smooth.

Remove donor punches using toothed forceps. A 5-inch, 2-to-1 Brown-Adson tooth-type forceps is used commonly. Grasp the plug on one side near the edge of the epidermis to avoid crushing the hair roots. Gentle traction with toothed forceps will ease the plugs out of place, and small scissors may be used to snip the attached subcutaneous fat from the bottom of the plug. Some surgeons apply traction to the plug, observe it with a magnifying loupe, and use scissors to detach the plug so that it contains only a small amount of fat below the "black dots." In this way, they trim the plug while detaching it from the scalp. Remember that the "black dots" are not the bottom of the papillae but are the pigmented portion of the hair that lies immediately above the root. Therefore, be sure that you have some yellow fat on the bottom of the plug below each hair follicle. This is another part of the procedure in which the vital parts can be transected easily, resulting in no or poor growth.

Place the plugs on wet saline gauze in a disposable plastic or sterile glass Petri dish, in rows of ten to facilitate counting (Fig 5–10). Some surgeons prefer to put the plugs into a test tube of saline solution, shake vigorously to dislodge spicules of hair, and pour the saline solution containing the plugs onto a sterilized stainless steel screen or mesh gauze. This helps separate plugs from detached hair spicules.

Trim excess fat and residual hair spicules using fine forceps, small scissors, and sometimes a magnifying visor. Some years ago, it was believed that the plugs would "take" better if most of the fat was trimmed. Although this is true with respect to large, full-thickness grafts, it is not important for these tiny composite grafts. Plugs are trimmed to remove galea and excess fat so that the donor plug fits better into the recipient area, rather than to enhance takes.

The most important aspect of the trimming procedure is to remove spicules of hair or hair shafts without attached roots from the circumference of the cylindrical plug. These bare hairs will set up foreign-body reaction and cause extra scar tissue, which may result in destruction of other viable hair follicles. In the trimming process, plugs are best handled with delicate 2-to-1 toothed forceps of the Brown-Adson type. Again, grasp the plugs at the edge near the epidermis to prevent crush injury to roots. Gradle or small-curved iris scissors are favored for trimming. Then place the cleaned plugs on gauze soaked with physiologic saline solution in another Petri dish. Again, maintain rows of five or ten plugs each to keep track of the number of plugs.

RECIPIENT AREA

The recipient holes are made with a punch 0.5 or 0.25 mm smaller in diameter than the donor punch. Some surgeons prefer the basic four-set technique (Fig 5–11). At the initial sitting, recipient sites (labeled 1 in Fig 5–11) are made and transplanted. Four weeks later, the circles (labeled 2) are cut and planted, and so on with the third and fourth sets.[4–7] This method theoretically provides a greater amount of blood to each plug to achieve the maximum number of hairs per plug. Fill-in sessions then are done on a freehand basis.

To insert plugs, grasp them with fine-toothed forceps near the epidermis at what will be the most frontal (anterior) portion when the plug grows. Push the plug in perpendicular to the scalp and let it automatically curve and slide into place. Attempting to insert plugs by paralleling the angle of the hole, although ultimately logical, results in difficulty in proper insertion. Plugs should lie exactly level with the surface of the scalp or should be pushed into the scalp below surface level and then brought back up to level with the scalp. This maneuver will expel any small amounts of blood or blood clots that have gath-

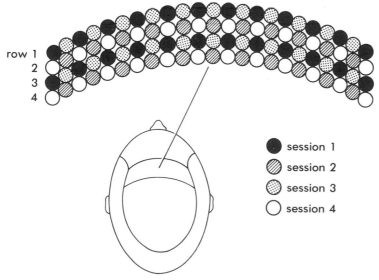

Fig 5–11.—Preplan for four sets of plugs.

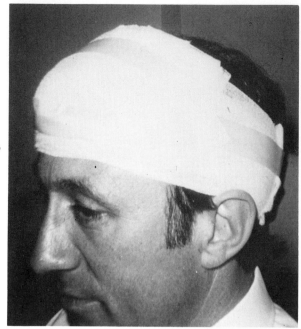

Fig 5–12.—Final head wrap covering both donor and recipient areas.

ered in the bottom of the recipient hole. If the angle of the hairs is not in the forward direction, rotate the plugs in place rather than taking them out and replacing them. Start with the most anterior row, insert the plugs, and then cover the inserted plugs with gauze and apply hand pressure while working on additional rows. This tends to set the plugs and provide hemostasis while the planting continues. A plug that tends to pop up is best set by wrapping the finger in gauze and applying pressure in a wiggling motion rather than trying to do it all with forceps. After all of the transplants are set, check the direction of hair growth on each plug and make minor adjustments by rotating the plugs.

When hemostasis is complete, no additional surgical attention need be paid to the recipient area. The patient now can leave with the head wrap previously wrapped around the donor and forehead areas, or a new, final wrap may be desired. The recipient area may be covered by Telfa dotted with antibiotic ointment and included in the final dressing (Fig 5–12). Although many patients believe that the recipient area should be bandaged, experience with both approaches has shown that it makes little difference in the final result. If the dressing is to be removed in the office the next day, the recipient area usually is covered. If the patient is to remove his own dressing, the recipient area usually is not covered, so the patient will not have the problem of removing the dressing and possibly pulling out the freshly planted plugs.

Postoperative bleeding almost never is a problem in the recipient area. Rarely, a recipient hole will have arterial bleeding sufficient to necessitate suturing. The recipient hole is closed, and another opening to accommodate the plug is cut. The sutured site can be transplanted at another time.

We do not use the basic four set but prefer to adapt the technique to the specific needs of the patient. To fill a wide frontal area, even a wide frontotemporal recession, we usually place the most posterior plugs at the first session

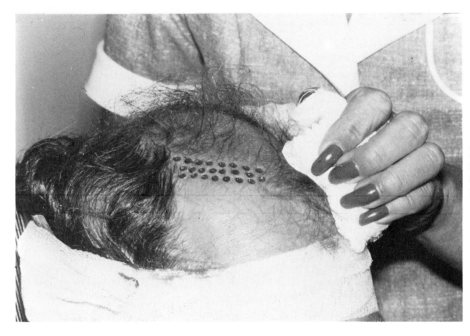

Fig 5–13.—Posterior portion of hairline done initially. Next session will place plugs (anteriorly) to determine actual frontal hairline.

(Fig 5–13). The recipient holes are separated from one another by a distance equal to or less than one plug's diameter. This allows blood supply to come around each plug, facilitates coverage of future transplants by existing or transplanted hair, and allows each set of plugs to have the full head of pressure from the arterial system. Although plugs are not always set in exact rows on the top or frontal area of the scalp, maximal hair growth is achieved when the equivalent of four rows or fewer are placed at one time. A fifth or sixth row

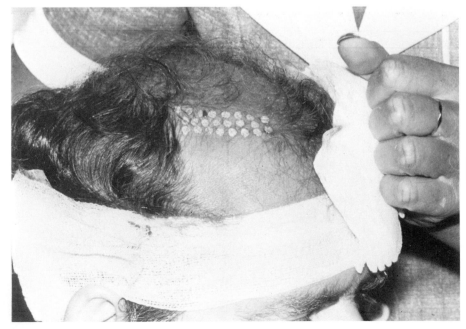

Fig 5–14.—Plugs placed so that less than one plug width exists between adjacent plugs.

posterior to the frontal row will grow, but with fewer hairs than the four anterior rows. A month later, more rows may be placed anteriorly to the first set in order to approach or make a frontal hairline.

Working from the midcrown toward the anterior hairline in successive transplant sessions allows each set of newly transplanted hairs to have the benefit of the full perfusion of the superficial temporal arterial system. Exact waiting times between transplant sessions vary with patients. Most conservative surgeons wait a month before placing new plugs between previously transplanted plugs. Under special circumstances, we have successfully transplanted on Monday, Wednesday, and Friday of the same week, placing approximately 250 plugs over the entire scalp. If this is done, any infection or other untoward effects could lead to loss of a massive amount of irreplaceable transplants. Most surgeons recommend doing fewer than 100 plugs per session and spreading these transplants over the greatest possible area of scalp to provide each plug with the greatest possible blood supply.

More important than the total number of plugs is the number of plugs planted per area. Certainly, 100 plugs crowded into one-fourth of the scalp area will give poor growth. The experienced surgeon will adjust the number of plugs to the size of the area transplanted to achieve the best growth and cosmetic result. Limit the frontal one-fourth of scalp to 50–70 plugs per session and limit the whole scalp to 100–150 plugs per session.

When making the hairline itself, place the initial plugs so that less than one plug width exists between adjacent plugs (Fig 5–14). If all plugs do not grow to their full circumference, a fill-in plug can be placed directly between two adjacent plugs. If, by good fortune, all of the hairs do grow, a fill-in plug can be placed slightly behind and abutting the original two plugs.

There are two approaches to cutting the frontal recipient holes. The first approach, generally followed by those using the basic four-set pattern, entails cutting the plug holes at an angle approximately 60 degrees to the frontal scalp (Fig 5–15). This 60-degree angle provides growth of hair with a higher look but

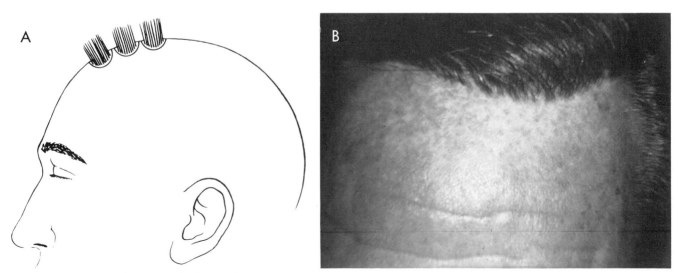

Fig 5–15.—A, 60-degree angle frontal hairline technique. **B,** clinical example showing higher growth of hair from the scalp.

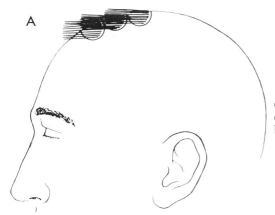

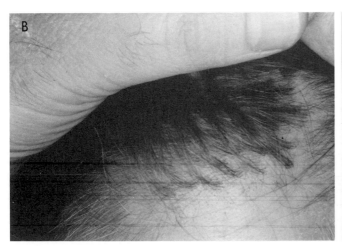

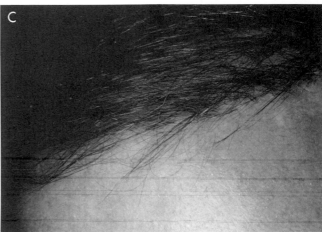

Fig 5–16.—**A,** 30-degree angle frontal hairline technique. **B,** clinical example with hair elevated to show relatively small number of plugs done thus far. **C,** automatic overlap giving flatter growth but thicker look with fewer plugs.

requires a greater number of plugs to provide a full look. In the second approach, the punch enters the scalp at an angle of 30 degrees or less. It is almost impossible to make this angle too acute. Plugs growing in will overlap one another to yield a shingling effect that automatically hides individual plugs and provides greater coverage with fewer plugs. The frontal hair will grow less high but will require fewer plugs to achieve a full look (Fig 5–16).

This approach is practical only when there is no residual hair in the area. When doing transplants for thinning hair, or if significant amounts of hair remain immediately adjacent to the transplanted area, the surgeon should cut the recipient holes exactly parallel to existing hairs to avoid cutting the roots of hairs adjacent to the transplanted area. The paralleling technique preserves hair that might never be lost and allows a fuller look. Which is better? The surgeon should know both techniques and use whichever is best for the individual patient.

Another consideration is the patients' combing method. If a side-to-side or side-to-front method is used, greater numbers of plugs should be placed on the parted side. This makes the part line and the side thicker, and those hairs combed sideways or forward contribute to a dense appearance of the other side.

POST TRANSPLANTS

We give the patients nonaspirin-containing pain medication such as codeine, 30 mg, with Tylenol or Percocet. Some patients will postpone filling prescriptions for pain medications immediately after surgery because the lidocaine is still in effect. The surgeon often gets a 1 A.M. phone call because the patient wants to know which pharmacy is open all night. The small cost of giving patients pain medication from an office supply has saved us many nights' sleep. Patients are told to take the pain medicine only if it is really necessary, that pain medicine often "works" quite well just being kept in the pocket, and that if they do not want to take the potent pain medicine we give them, they should take nonaspirin-containing medications such as Tylenol or Datril to avoid aspirin-induced bleeding. Often the same pain pills resting on the patient's nightstand provide excellent relief from pain for several transplant sessions.

Ideally, the patient returns to the office the next day for removal of the bandage; removal of the Gelfoam layers, if used; and for cleaning of any dried blood with peroxide, aqueous Zephiran, or Hibiclens. In practice, most patients remove the bandage themselves and gently clean the desired area with peroxide, cotton-tipped applicators, and soap and water or a Water Pik. The patient then combs the hair, being careful to comb the hair high off the scalp in the recipient area to avoid hooking a plug with the comb. Hair spray may be used the morning after hair transplantation to hold hair in place and so disguise the recipient area. Shampooing is permitted three days after the hair transplant session, with the recipient area being cleansed initially as follows: a washcloth is wet and shampoo is lathered into it. This soapy washcloth is laid over the recipient area and the shower water is allowed to beat on the washcloth, thus cleansing the recipient area by a leeching action. Rubbing the recipient area is not permitted for one week. Patients are told that if they try, they can pull recipient plugs out during the first week but that after two weeks, we cannot pull plugs out even by grasping them with forceps. Prophylactic antibiotics are not generally used except in special circumstances or if the patient

Fig 5–17.—Usual configuration of frontal hairline. Note hairline is in a C-shape, with no plugs planted in the temporal areas.

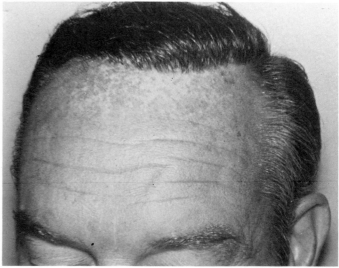

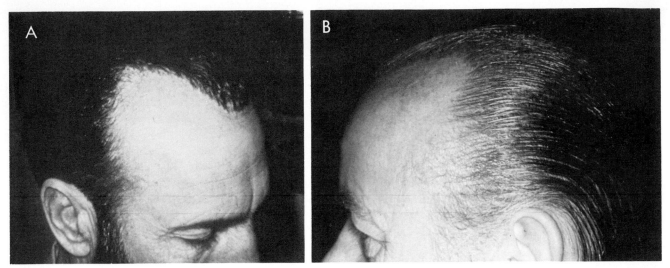

Fig 5–18.—A, deep recession extended S-shaped hairline for older patients or patients with limited numbers of plugs. **B,** same. Note that fine plugs may need to be placed judiciously in the temporal area.

is greatly concerned. In these cases, it is best to start antibiotic therapy immediately on arrival of the patient in the office, before starting the transplant procedure. Medication should be continued for one to two days in standard dosages. Infection is relatively uncommon. Minoxidil 2% solution applied topically daily to transplants probably enhances growth of hair or retards telogen loss.

PLANNING THE HAIRLINE

Most patients will be given a C-shaped hairline (Fig 5–17). Older patients will receive the deep recession extended S-shaped curve (Fig 5–18). Remember that approximately 75 plugs are necessary to lower the frontal hairline 1.0 cm. Therefore, the deeply recessed extended S curve may be beneficial for individ-

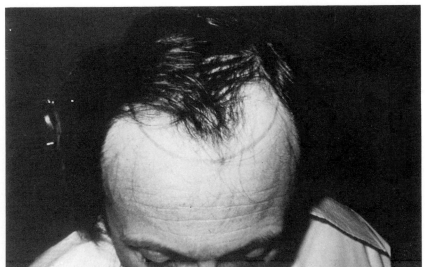

Fig 5–19.—Drawing of typical C-shaped hairline. Temporal recessions are always planned to give more natural look.

uals with limited donor sites. We draw the hairline on the patient's head and have the patient review it with us (Fig 5–19). We explain that although the hairline looks a little high when drawn with a felt marker, the effective visual hairline is significantly lower, since the hair grows forward. Additional rows or parts of the hairline always can be added. We explain that the hairline of a 28-year-old will look much better over the years than the hairline of a 16-year-old. We allow patient input into selection of the hairline but do not allow patients to talk us into juvenile hairlines.

Although we can say with certainty that transplants have lasted for 20 to 25 years, we believe that they will last a lifetime and must consider how the patients will look at various stages in their lifetime. Most remedial work in hair transplantation is done because hairlines were placed too low or temporal recessions were totally filled in, creating an inappropriate hairline for the adult lifetime.

In general 4.5-mm plugs are transplanted into 4.0-mm holes. For better blending, 4.0-mm plugs are used in the 3.5-mm holes. For fill-ins in the front row, 3.5-mm, 3.0-mm, 2.5-mm, or 2.0-mm plugs are transplanted into 0.5-mm smaller holes. We believe that the density in the anterior 2.0 cm is more important than a regular or irregular pattern. Placing a plug here and there in the front of the main body of transplanted hair to give a more natural appearance only gives the appearance of a plug placed here and there in front of the main transplanted hair mass. Transplanting individual hairs, using a trocar to create the recipient site, gives a natural appearance. The hairs are obtained from the sides of regular plugs. Planting 20–50 individual hairs per side, one can soften the plug effect of the hairline. Details of this technique will be published by Emanuel Marritt in the near future. Density in the first 2.0 cm is most important, whether it is achieved by hair plugs of a variety of sizes set close together or by a shingling technique.

"Micrografts," recently described by Rolf Nordstrom,[8] essentially transplant groups of three hairs into the leading edge of the frontal hairline. These provide filling in between adjacent circular plugs, help disguise cobblestoning and sharp color differences, and soften a hairline composed of coarse hairs.

Four-millimeter donor plugs containing the diameter of hairs desired are taken from the lower occipital region where small-diameter hairs are available. These circular plugs are cut longitudinally with iris scissors or microsurgery scissors, using magnification. Each 4.0-mm plug provides three to five micrografts containing two to four hairs. Small incisions about 3.0 mm long and 4.0 mm apart which may penetrate the galea aponeurotica are made with a #11 blade. The micrografts are inserted with jewelers' forceps or microsurgical forceps by grasping at one epidermal edge or by pulling them in place by the fat that was left below the follicles specifically for this purpose. Remember, the papillae are below the black dots seen, so that sufficient fat must be present to prevent crush injury of the hair roots. The tops of the micrografts are left level with or below the surrounding epidermis. Repeated micrograft sessions can be done every two weeks. Usually two or three sessions are required.

The best frontal hairline effect comes from the combination of repeated fill-in sessions and appropriate advice on hair styling (Fig 5–20 to 5–24).

The same general techniques are used for congenital or traumatic defects, thermal burns, surgical scars, androgenic alopecia in women, and alopecia secondary to burned-out diseases. Plugs have been placed under split-thickness

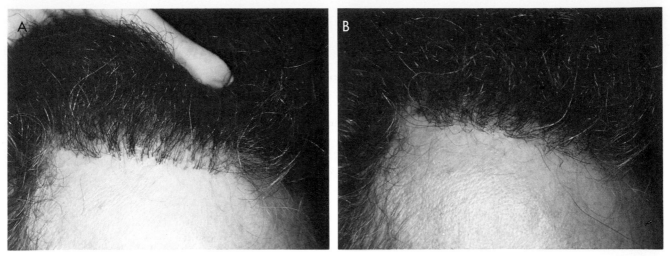

Fig 5–20.—A, hairline of plugs exposed by lifting. **B,** hairline in normal social situation.

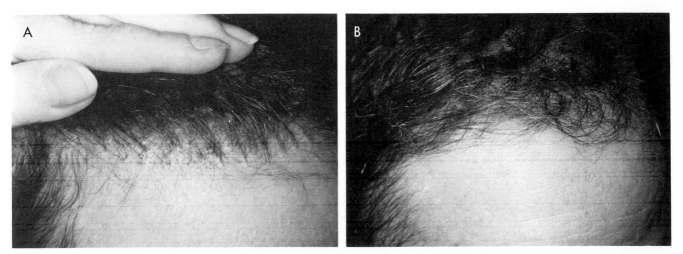

Fig 5–21.—A, frontal hairline plugs exposed. **B,** hairline in normal social situation.

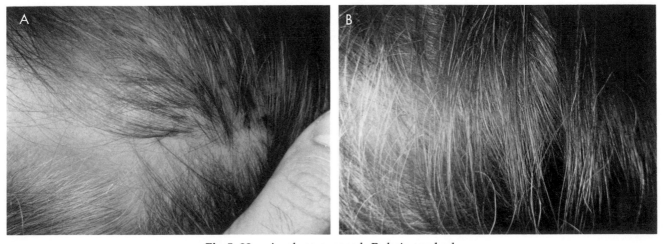

Fig 5–22.—A, plugs exposed. **B,** hair combed.

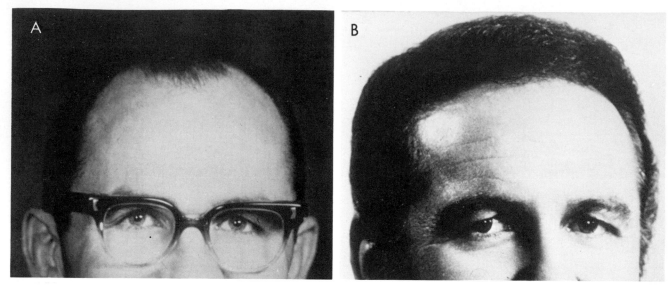

Fig 5–23.—A, prior to transplants. **B,** after transplants.

grafts, but we have not had the opportunity to do this. In scar tissue, fewer hairs per plug will grow, with 50%–75% of the normal amount being the rule. When transplanting alopecia secondary to burned-out disease, we wait a year or more after all disease activity has ceased and appreciate that even with this conservative approach, the old disease might be reactivated.

COMPLICATIONS

A variety of complications occurs with the punch graft method. Fortunately, when proper technique is followed, almost all of the complications are minor and easily handled in the office.

There are the general complications seen with any type of skin surgery. Bleeding from the donor site is uncommon and from the recipient site is rare. It may occur when the epinephrine effect of the local anesthetic wears off, 4–6 hours postoperatively. Use of the suture techniques and the head wrap, and teaching the patient that pressure usually stops the bleeding result in rare occurrences of postoperative bleeding requiring attention. We average one night call from our transplant patients about every six months. Bleeding in the donor area is handled by one interrupted or figure eight suture. Bleeding in the recipient area is handled by an interrupted suture and replacement of that plug in a nearby recipient area.

Infection occurs in fewer than 1% of patients. It is managed by oral erythromycin, tetracycline, or a semisynthetic penicillin. We have seen only a few serious infections. We had one infection due to *Pseudomonas,* which was the result of the overzealous use of hexachlorophene shampoo by the patient before the transplants.

Edema is expected. Transplanting more than 30 plugs per session in the front commonly results in swelling of the forehead, usually on the third to fifth day. This is edema fluid being pulled by gravity from the recipient site. As the edema fluid drifts in its plane into eyelid tissue, black eyes may result. This is

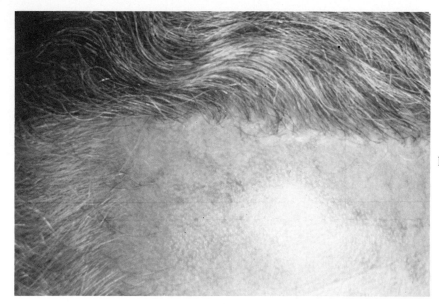

Fig 5–24.—Frontal hairline. Patient previously completely bald on top.

self-limiting, but we always warn patients of the possibility so they will not be alarmed by it. Application of ice packs immediately after transplantation and continued at home the first day may be preventive. We have not found steroids to be helpful.

The Koebner phenomenon is seen, particularly in psoriasis. Patients who have active psoriasis, especially of the scalp, should be warned that psoriasis may develop around the transplanted hair. This is treated by the usual antipsoriatic measures.

Complications specific for the donor area include foreign-body reaction, arteriovenous (AV) fistulas, large scars, and painful scars. Foreign-body reactions most likely are due to hair spicules being sewn into the wound. They are rare, with an incidence of less than 1% and are managed by injection of triamcinolone 4 mg/ml or with appropriate incision and drainage. Single painful scars may occur; their exact cause is not known. Generally, injection with triamcinolone, 4 mg/ml, solves the problem. In unusual cases, punch excision of that particular scar with or without suture closure solves the problem. The patient may have had 200 plugs taken and have one painful scar. Large scar areas result from taking plugs too closely and not leaving enough intervening skin and blood supply to support hair growth between donor sites. Taking plugs one plug width apart prevents this problem, as does the Pierce method of closure. Taking too many plugs close together in a vertical direction can produce excess thinning so that the hair parts and shows the scar. Correction is with proper styling or excision of scar tissue to bring the hairy edges together.

Complications of the recipient area include alteration in the color of the skin. In some patients who have been bald for a long time, the frontal scalp is a darker color owing to sun exposure compared with the whiter skin of the recipient area, which has been covered by a blanket of hair. This white donor skin can be noticed particularly before the hair grows. Usually, the continued outdoor activity of the patient causes the color to even out over two to three years.

Another group of people will develop white rings around the plugs or lose all pigment in the plug itself. These people inherently lose pigment with any sort of trauma to their skin. A patient who has white linear surgical scars or white spots from liquid nitrogen treatment should be advised of this possibility. The solution is hairstyling. Pigment cells may regrow into those areas after many, many years, but permanent depigmentation may result. Fortunately, the observing eye generally sees the hair that is growing and does not focus on the hypopigmented skin. Proper styling is a necessary part of hair transplantation.

Cobblestoning or elevation of transplanted plugs almost always is due to the inherent healing features of the patient. It is seen in patients who are prone to hypertrophic scar formation. We have purposely planted donor plugs depressed below the skin level, elevated above the skin level, and at skin level. Within the limits of our experience, we have not found a consistent difference in the results. Obviously, one should try to place the plugs level with the skin surface, but during the healing process, the plugs level out. The single best treatment for elevated plugs, whether one or two plugs in the frontal hairline or a feature of almost all the plugs of the frontal hairline, is to use the epilating needle on an electrocoagulation machine. The epilating needle destroys excess elevated surface tissue without affecting the hair. This allows the patient to be treated but retain the number of hairs and hairstyle before treatment. Use of dermabrasion, shave techniques, or hot cautery necessitate that hairs be cut and the patient goes through a period of cosmetic disfigurement. Although a superficial thermal burn is produced by the epilation needle, we have not seen this result in hypertrophic scarring. In our hands it is the ideal method.

The commonest side effects are associated with the growth of hair itself. The most serious problem is failure to grow. The commonest causes are cutting off the hair roots when removing the donor plug or cutting off the roots when trimming the donor plugs. Each plug must contain sufficient fat to be sure roots are included. We are aware of one case described at a medical meeting in which the patient had four test plugs. Each plug became red and the hair failed to grow. A few months later, four more test plugs were done with the same reddening and failure to grow. Transplantation was not continued further. This is the only case of this type of which we are aware. An occasional plug may be lost owing to Valsalva's maneuvers during exercise or straining during the first few days posttransplantation.

Variations in growth occur. Most patients will show early growth by ten weeks with growth noticeable to the patient by three months. However, doing large numbers of plugs, e.g., 200 or more, can delay growth for six months. Doing too many plugs can result in central scalp slough, as occurred in a case report in which more than 600 plugs were done at one session. Prevention is simply to do smaller numbers—e.g., 50–100 plugs—and to spread them over a greater area. In some patients the initial growth is kinky or wiry. In almost all patients this kind of growth reverts to normal within two years. Hair growing in the wrong direction generally is due to plugs having been planted in the wrong direction. Some plugs will grow fewer hairs than others. Sometimes this is due to chance. Other times it can be anticipated; for example, the fifth row and beyond from the frontal line consistently grow fewer hairs than the first four rows. It is assumed that the scar tissue inhibits blood flow. If possible, prevention is to do the more posterior rows first and allow those plugs to establish themselves with maximal growth. Then do the more frontal rows. Variation in growth between two sides on an individual is common. We have seen some individuals who consistently have 50% more hairs per plug on one side of the scalp than on the other no matter what the donor area plug size or technique used. Sometimes a patient will complain that the plugs done by his previous physician grew more hair than your plugs. Use of different-sized donor plugs or even the same size made by different manufacturers, as described above, can be a factor. Also, the first physician may have been putting plugs into scalp without scar, and your fill-in plugs might go into areas where scar tissue exists from prior transplantation. This can lower the yield of hairs.

An occasional patient will complain of the "bush effect." Rather than doing epilation to decrease the number of hairs, it generally is more effective to add additional grafts to try to get a dense, 2.0-cm band of frontal hair by using regular-sized plugs or micrografts described above. Patients may jokingly complain that you transplanted gray hair to the front. Most people do not appreciate how much gray hair they have in the back. We know of a single case in which gray and black hair transplanted from the back grew as all black hair.

The commonest problem of hairline placement is the straight frontal hairline, which usually is done by less experienced hair transplanters. The treatment is to remove the low plugs and suture close or replace the low plugs with hairless adjacent scalp skin. With the advent of scalp reduction, excessively high lateral frontal hairlines may be seen. The experienced hair transplanter deliberately will place the hairline much lower so that it looks abnormally low. Repeated scalp reduction then raises the lateral hairline into the proper position. This requires experience, since the amount of bald scalp to be reduced varies with the patient as well as the variety of scalp reduction techniques that can be used.

After transplantation has started, some patients decide they do not want the hair transplants because "it's not them." Repeated epilation can rid the hairs but the difference in skin will persist. The best solution is to find out psychologically what bothers these patients about the plugs. The solution is almost always to add additional plugs to give them a thicker look or to refer them to a good hair stylist. Elliptical or punch excisions to remove the transplants are possible but are generally less satisfactory.

Patients return years later with additional hair loss. They may show an island of hair transplants. Extension of the hairlines to join the receding hair and plug fill-ins solves the problem. Additional loss of hair should be contemplated at the time of doing the initial plugs. For example, when reducing the temporal recession with the plugs, the two side hairlines should be planned so that it will be easy to connect them and make a continuous hairline someday when the midfrontal hair is lost. We must plan to adjust the transplanted area over the lifetime of the patient.

Occurrence of AV fistulas probably produces the most anxiety in the beginning hair transplanter. These most commonly occur in the donor area and increase in incidence when plugs greater than 4.5 mm are taken. The patient notices a swelling or a pulsating swelling in the back of the head. Sometimes this results in a large, relatively thick-walled aneurysm. Most AV fistulas spontaneously disappear, although it seems wise to treat them all. The simplest treatment is to inject triamcinolone acetonide 4–10 mg/ml around the aneurysm, taking care not to inject intravascularly. It has not been possible to do controlled studies, but the resolution of the AV fistula seems to occur more rapidly with this treatment than with spontaneous resolution.

The next easiest treatment is to define the afferent arterial flow by finger palpation. A percutaneous suture of 0 silk, Vicryl or Dexon can be placed through the skin, beneath the vessel, out the skin and tied tightly. Shutting off arterial inflow solves the problem. If these methods are not effective or if the skin and aneurysm appear to be thinning, simple surgical removal in the office is the definitive approach. Very careful incision over or immediately adjacent to the aneurysm, followed by blunt dissection will define the aneurysmal sac along with the enlarged arteriole and vein. Double ligatures of 3-0 Vicryl, Dexon, or permanent suture are applied and the mass removed. Careful skin closure results in a narrow scar, well hidden by the hair.

More annoying are AV fistulas in the recipient area. These fortunately are quite rare but will cause an enlargement and prominence of the branch of the superficial temporal artery feeding the fistula. Pulsating forehead sensations are felt, and some patients will have severe vascular headaches. Treatment is the same as for AV fistula of the donor area. The only one we have seen was solved with a percutaneous suture. If excision is necessary, the placement of the scar that will result is most important.

Although the side effects and complications of hair transplants may be numerous, they fortunately are readily handled by simple techniques that can be performed in any well-equipped office.

REFERENCES

1. Orentreich N.: Autografts in alopecias and other selected dermatological conditions. *Ann. N.Y. Acad. Sci.* 83:463–479, 1959.
2. Orentreich N.: Hair transplants, in Maddin S. (ed.): *Current Dermatologic Therapy.* St. Louis, C.V. Mosby Co., 1975, pp. 26–32.
3. Hagerman O., Wilson J.: The skin biopsy punch: Evaluation and modification. *Cutis* 6:1139–1143, 1970.
4. Unger W.P.: *Hair Transplantation.* New York, Marcel Dekker, 1978.
5. Norwood O.T.: *Hair Transplant Surgery.* Springfield, Ill., Charles C Thomas Publisher, 1973.
6. Ayres S. III: Hair transplantation, in Epstein E., and Epstein E. Jr. (eds.): *Skin Surgery.* Springfield, Ill., Charles C Thomas Publisher, 1982.
7. Vallis C.T.: *Hair Transplantation for the Treatment of Male Pattern Baldness.* Springfield, Ill., Charles C Thomas Publisher, 1982.
8. Nordstrom R.E.A.: Micrografts for improvement of the frontal hairline after hair transplantation. *Aesth. Plast. Surg.* 5:97–101, 1981.

6 / Strip Grafts for Alopecia

STRIP GRAFTS WERE pioneered by Charles Vallis, whose first publication was in 1969.[1,2] At that time, the punch autograft technique was relatively new and not sophisticated enough to produce the kinds of results that are considered standard today. It was common to have a brush-like appearance with transplant plugs. This was particularly true on the frontal hairline, where there would be a plug of hair, a space, a plug of hair, a space, and so on. Vallis reasoned that a long strip of hair taken from the occipital region would produce a smoother and more normal-looking hairline. After various trials, he developed the Vallis strip graft handle, which consisted of a scalpel handle with two #15 blades attached in parallel (Fig 6–1). The distance between the blades could be set with various shims. Usually a 5.0- to 6.0-mm width is used because this produces a strip that is most consistent with good hair growth. When exceeding a 6.0-mm width, hair growth in some individuals is excellent, but in many others the central portion often does not grow. Some strips up to 9.0 mm wide have been successful, but generally Vallis recommends a 6.0-mm strip for the most satisfactory results.[3,4]

TECHNIQUE (FIG 6–2)

The scalp is prepared in the same way as for hair transplants, which involves shampooing the hair the morning of or the night before surgery with an anti-

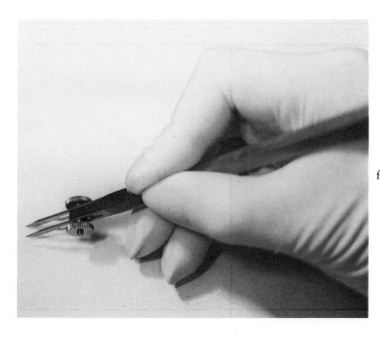

Fig 6–1.—Vallis double-bladed scalpel for taking strip grafts.

Fig 6–2.—A, taking donor strip, using Vallis scalpel. **B,** removing hair strip with scissors. **C,** strip removed from donor site. **D,** donor site sutured.

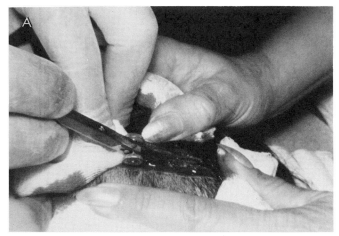

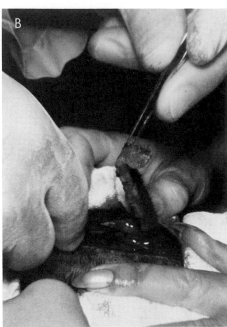

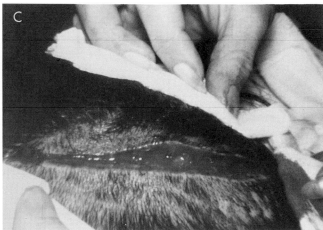

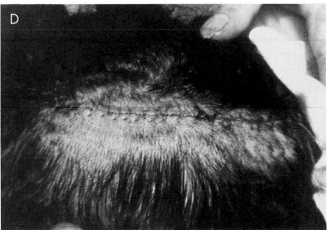

bacterial shampoo. The posterior scalp hair is lifted, and a segment of the scalp hair is trimmed to approximately ⅛ in. long. The desired frontal hairline is drawn. A string, suture, gauze, or other malleable substance is used to take an exact measurement of the length needed and of the curve of the proposed frontal hairline. This length then is marked off on the donor occipital area, and an extra 10%–25% length is added to allow for the contraction of a full-thickness skin graft when it is excised free from its bed.

Anesthesia is obtained with lidocaine 1% with epinephrine 1:100,000. The Vallis strip handle is used to cut from one end of the donor area to the other, being extremely careful to angle the blades so that they are parallel to the long axis of the hairs (Fig 6–2,A). This, of course, assumes that the hair roots are in the same axial line. Failure to line up the hairs perfectly will result in poor hair growth. The Vallis scalpel is drawn slowly and carefully over the length of the

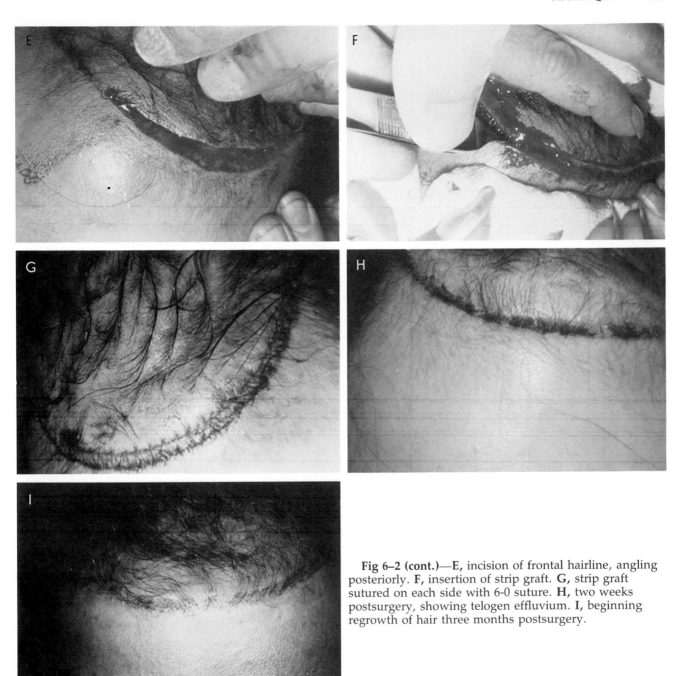

Fig 6–2 (cont.)—E, incision of frontal hairline, angling posteriorly. **F,** insertion of strip graft. **G,** strip graft sutured on each side with 6-0 suture. **H,** two weeks postsurgery, showing telogen effluvium. **I,** beginning regrowth of hair three months postsurgery.

donor line. In most cases, the blades do not completely cut through the skin, so a regular #15 blade on the normal scalpel handle is used to complete the cut to the desired depth into the fat.

The strip is removed very carefully with small forceps or skin hooks. The base of the attaching fat must be cut with scissors (Fig 6–2,B and C). It is placed in normal saline solution for holding. During the incision and excision process, the assistant must press firmly above and below the donor area to keep the field relatively free from blood. Failure to have a good assistant makes this procedure far more difficult than it need be. Hemostasis is obtained by electro-coagulation; rarely, a bleeder must be ligated with suture (Fig 6–2,D). The donor area is closed with a running suture such as 3-0 Mersilene or, if there is a great deal of tension, a 2-0 or 0 Prolene or nylon is used. There is no need to bury any sutures. A snug and properly placed running suture not only brings the edges together but also achieves good hemostasis.

For the frontal hairline, a regular-handled #15 blade is used to incise the frontal scalp. The incision is made slowly and carefully over the whole length of the previously drawn frontal hairline, being careful to angle the cut 45 degrees in a posterior direction (Fig 6–2,E). Since the hairs in the occipital area are growing in an inferior or caudad angle at approximately 45 degrees, matching this angle of the incision in front is necessary to provide a smooth fit and make a more natural-looking frontal hairline. Most of the time when the frontal hairline is incised through the skin completely, it will gape wider than 6.0 mm. If it does not gape this much, the incision should be carried through the galea and the incision line will easily open wide enough to accommodate the graft. Again, hemostasis is obtained with electrocoagulation.

The strip of hair is examined with magnification. It should show that almost all of the hair shafts are complete, from the stubble of hair through the hair root and hair bulb. Any free shafts not attached to the root should be snipped off with scissors.

The strip is placed into the wound on the anterior scalp so that the hair is aimed forward in the normal growth pattern for that area (Fig 6–2,F). The strip is sutured anteriorly and posteriorly with a running 6-0 nylon or 6-0 Prolene suture on a P-1 or P-3 needle, being careful to control how much of the strip graft itself is encompassed in each suture (Fig 6–2,G). Only the edge of the strip should be caught in the loop of the suture so that no blood supply in the center portion of the graft is compromised. Other suture techniques are acceptable, but it is important to remember not to strangulate the center portion of the graft with the sutures.

A moderate amount of pressure is applied through a pressure dressing utilizing a head wrap with Kerlix or similar materials. Sutures can be removed in a week if healing is progressing satisfactorily.

The hairs go into telogen phase, and for three or four weeks following the procedure the hairs will progressively fall out until none are left (Fig 6–2,H). The patient should be advised that the telogen resting phase is normal and that if all goes well and the graft is sufficiently nourished, a full 6.0-mm width of the strip will begin growing between three and six months after the surgical procedure.

The advantage of this technique is that a smooth, even hairline, 5.0–6.0 mm wide can be obtained without the bunching or brush look seen with punch autografts (Fig 6–3). A negative feature of the technique is that the observing eye seems to look deeper through the frontal hairline than 5.0–6.0 mm and can see the stripping effect with the thin or bald hair behind (Fig 6–4,A–C). This phenomenon can be tested on oneself by looking in a mirror and using a yellow lead pencil placed between the hairs at various distances from the frontal

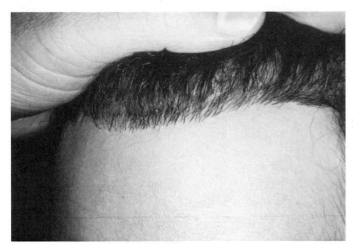

Fig 6–3.—Excellent frontal hairline created by strip graft.

hairline. You will notice that if the pencil is placed closer to the frontal hairline than 1.5–2.0 cm, it is clearly noticed. Only posterior to that distance is it hidden by the hairs.

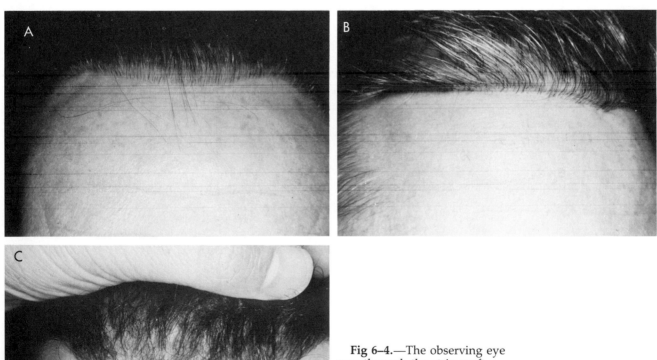

Fig 6–4.—The observing eye sees through the strip graft.

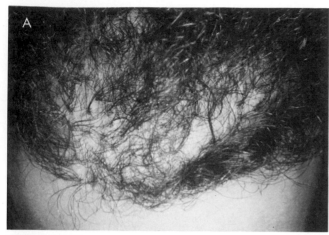

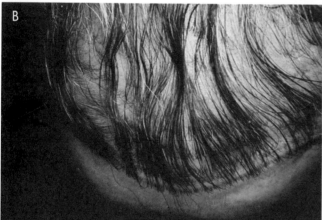

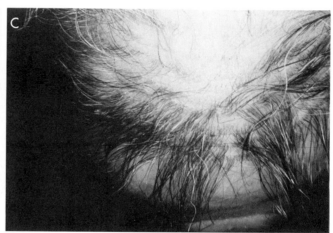

Fig 6–5.—A, plugs needed behind frontal strip graft for fill-in. **B,** additional strips placed behind frontal strip graft hairline for fill-in. **C,** strips placed throughout scalp, showing technical difficulty of joining them into one hair mass.

Consequently, additional hair must be placed behind the strip, with either hair plugs (Fig 6–5,A) or additional strips (Fig 6–5,B). The bald scalp between the strips may need to be excised; however, complete apposition of several of these small strips generally is not successful because of the difficulty of excising long, narrow, curved areas of bald scalp without removing any of the newly planted strip (Fig 6–5,C). Most surgeons use hair plugs behind the strips.

One of the commonest errors made with strip grafts is that the surgeon will try to cut the graft freehand with a single #15 or #10 blade. After the initial cut is made on one side of the strip, it is quite difficult to make a smooth, even second cut 6.0 mm away. For a strip of skin that is only 5.0–6.0 mm wide, any waviness or variation, with resultant loss of thickness of the strip, is an extremely serious error. We all need to take into account that Vallis, who developed this technique and did many of the strips, felt the need to develop a special instrument and highly recommends it for acceptable results. We should take heed from his experience.

Because his original technique gave a sharply defined hairline, Vallis developed another instrument consisting of two corrugated metal pieces with one edge of each sharpened. These fit together to cut a hair strip with a built-in irregularity to better simulate the irregularity of the normal hairline. After preparation of the donor site as described above, the sharp edges are pressed into the donor area, removed, and pressed in again immediately adjacent to the first site. By repeating the process, a strip of the desired length with an irregular edge can be prepared. A #15 scalpel blade is used to cut through the deep dermis into the fat so the strip can be removed. The remainder of the procedure is as described above. Whether this instrument gives a sufficiently normal-looking hairline depends on individual judgment.

For selected patients, with careful attention to details of the technique, as described in Vallis's articles and book, hair strips provide one more modality for achieving correction of male pattern alopecia.

EYEBROW REPLACEMENT

The original Vallis double-bladed scalpel can be used to take short strips for replacement of lost eyebrows (Fig 6–6,A–D). Although these can be taken freehand, the Vallis instrument can provide more even widths of strips. It is most important to remember that strips taken for eyebrow replacement should be taken superior-inferior—i.e., cephalad-caudad—in contrast to strips taken for

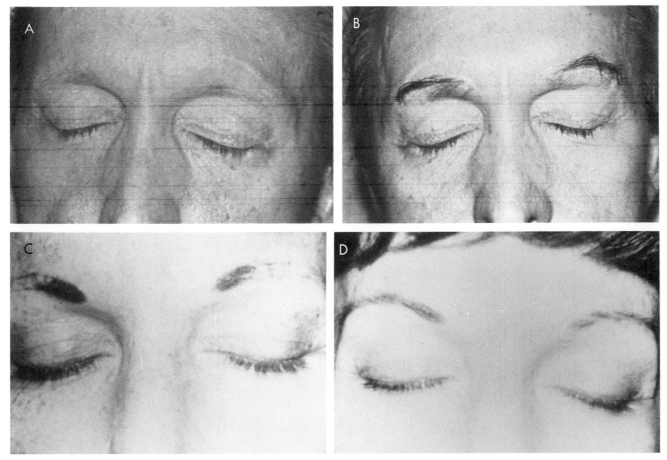

Fig 6–6.—**A,** absence of eyebrows. **B,** strip grafts placed. **C,** absence of lateral portions of eyebrows. **D,** strip grafts growing. (Courtesy of Leonard Lewis, M.D., Miami.)

scalp hairlines. If thinner hairs are desired for the lateral portion of the eyebrow, the strip can be taken partly off the neck where these finer hairs naturally occur. Taking strips in the up-down direction provides automatic overlap of hair in a progressive lateral direction as normally occurs in eyebrows.

In replacing permanently lost or congenitally absent eyebrows using the strip technique, the site and shape of the new eyebrow is carefully drawn on the patient. The proper length and curve of the eyebrows varies among patients and so the patient must be part of the planning process to insure a happier result. The eyebrow length and width should be drawn and agreed upon before lidocaine with epinephrine is injected and alters the area. The selected width of scalp hair is taken with the Vallis double scalpel from the occipital area in the cephalad-caudad direction, taking 10%–25% extra length to account for contraction when the strip is removed. For long eyebrows a second strip may need to be taken. The donor site(s) is closed with 3-0 Mersilene, while the donor strip rests in saline solution in a Petri dish. Hair shafts without roots are removed with scissors and excess nonhair bearing skin trimmed away.

The eyebrows are incised along the predetermined line. Sufficient gaping of skin occurs to allow insertion of the strip(s), so that the hairs overlap in a lateral direction. The strip(s) are sutured along each length using 6-0 Prolene on a P-3 or P-1 needle or a similar fine suture. Sutures are removed in a week. The hairs will go into telogen effluvium over the next 3–4 weeks. Regrowth of new hair begins in 2½–3 months. Once hairs are growing, the final shape of the eyebrow can be determined and maintained by routine plucking.

Similarly, good results can be obtained with the punch graft technique, utilizing 4.5-mm punches for the medial portion of the eyebrow and using smaller punches as one progresses laterally. Again, the angle of the punches must be acute to the skin's surface so that adjacent punches will overlap, producing the natural growth pattern of the eyebrow.

REFERENCES

1. Vallis C.P.: Surgical treatment of the receding hairline. *Plast. Reconstr. Surg.* 44:271–278, 1969.
2. Vallis C.P.: Hair transplantation for male pattern baldness. *Surg. Clin. North Am.* 51:519–531, 1971.
3. Vallis C.P. in Rees T.D. (ed.): *Aesthetic Plastic Surgery.* New York, W.B. Saunders, 1980, p. 885.
4. Vallis C.P.: *Hair Transplantation for the Treatment of Male Pattern Alopecia.* Springfield, Ill., Charles C Thomas Publisher, 1982, pp. 189–281.

7 / Scalp Reduction for Alopecia

THE FIRST PAPER on scalp reduction published in English was in 1977 by Blanchard and Blanchard.[1] They reported 100 cases in which serial segments of bald skin had been removed from the scalp. Their procedure was called "hair lifting." They previously reported the technique in 1976 in the French literature.[2] In February 1978, at the International Hair Transplant Symposium in Lucerne, Switzerland, Stough and Webster, Sparkuhl, and the Blanchards all presented similar work, and there was extensive discussion on removal of bald skin as a treatment for male pattern alopecia.[3, 4] Although "hair lifting," "scalp reduction," and "alopecia reduction" all have been suggested as a name for the procedure, "scalp reduction" seems to be the one that is most widespread. This clearly was a surgical innovation that came at the right time. Physicians who had been doing hair transplants for many years seized on it as an excellent addition to the surgical modalities available for treatment of male pattern alopecia. Hair transplants have been quite successful, but if there was one area where they were least successful it was the posterior crown. There also was the inherent problem of an inadequate number of donors to completely fill the bald recipient area. This procedure seemed to partially meet both of these deficiencies in the standard hair transplant technique. The procedure has been refined in several ways since the initial presentation in 1977 and 1978, and there actually are some men whose baldness has been completely reduced by serial excisions.[5–9]

Although there are several scalp reduction procedures, the simplest is the midline sagittal scalp reduction (Figs 7–1 and 7–2). The procedure for this design is discussed in detail, followed by other designs and the rationale for choosing each of them.

TECHNIQUE

The patient is sedated if necessary. We tend to use little sedation, since our belief is that the fewer the medications, the fewer the problems. The patient can be sitting upright in a barber-type chair or can lie prone on the operating table. An ellipse, the length of the bald area and between 2.0 and 3.0 cm wide, is drawn. This ellipse does not extend farther anteriorly than the proposed transplanted frontal hairline. Actually, the tip of the ellipse should be 5.0 to 10.0 mm posterior to this proposed line. The posterior tip of the ellipse can extend to the posterior edge of the baldness and even into the miniaturizing hairs, which obviously are going to be lost in the ensuing years. The width is determined by manually testing the looseness of the scalp. If several furrows can be created in a midline plane by pushing the scalp together, 3.0 cm should be drawn in the initial ellipse. If the scalp feels tight, one might start with a 2.0-cm-wide ellipse.

Fig 7–1.—A, injection of lidocaine with epinephrine to produce field block of entire area of possible undermining and infiltration into lines of excision for hemostasis. **B,** incision of one side of ellipse and hemostasis. **C,** minimal area of undermining.

The scalp is cleansed with either Hibiclens or alcohol, and 1% Xylocaine with epinephrine 1:100,000 is injected circumferentially along the edges of what will be the maximal area of undermining, usually well within hair-bearing skin. The purpose of the first injection is to obtain a field block for the top of the head which will allow wide undermining without feeling. After this anesthesia has been placed, a second anesthesia is placed painlessly into the previously drawn lines of the ellipse (see Fig 7–1,A). The purpose of the second injection is to achieve deeper anesthesia and vasoconstriction at the incision site. It might be helpful to have stereo headphones, a TV, or stereo in the operatory because the most disconcerting part of the surgery to the patient is the sound of the undermining.

One side only of the ellipse is incised through the galea. Hemostasis is obtained with electrocautery or electrodesiccation (see Fig 7–1,B). It is helpful to have one or two assistants and suction. The edges of the scalp are everted, which allows the surgeon to desiccate those few large vessels quickly and easily. The bleeders are at the level of the galea and the deep dermal plexus. They are easy to see, and by obtaining hemostasis with this simple method, the entire procedure is easier to perform, particularly with the patient in the sitting position.

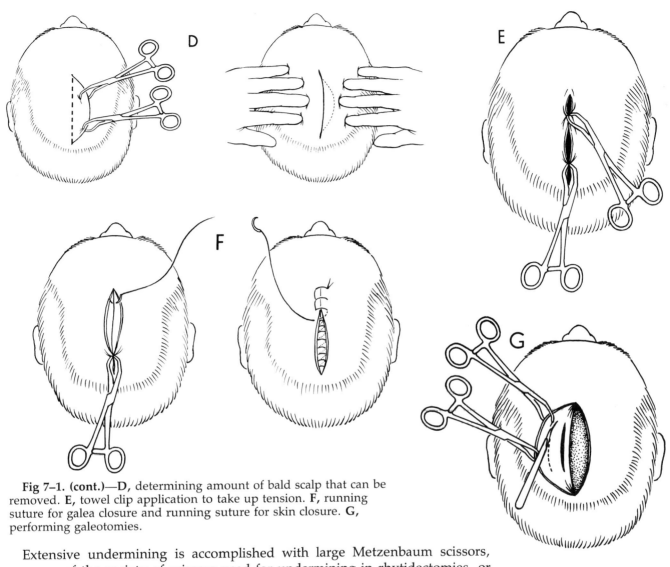

Fig 7–1. (cont.)—D, determining amount of bald scalp that can be removed. **E,** towel clip application to take up tension. **F,** running suture for galea closure and running suture for skin closure. **G,** performing galeotomies.

Extensive undermining is accomplished with large Metzenbaum scissors, any one of the variety of scissors used for undermining in rhytidectomies, or the Iconoclast, an undermining instrument developed by Ralph Luikart (see chap. 14). Minimal undermining is that of the whole top of the scalp (see Fig 7–1,C); maximal undermining would carry the undermining to the proposed anterior hairline, to the level of the ears, and to the lambdoid ridge. It is important to undermine below the galea because this is where there is the least amount of bleeding. Occasionally, there are some perforators, but most of the time there is just a thin fibrous stroma between the galea and the calvarium.

When the undermining is completed, the surgeon and assistant push or pull the scalp toward the midline so that the sides of the incised scalp overlap. With this maneuver, which can be accomplished with the fingers, skin hooks, forceps, or towel clips, it is easy to estimate the amount of bald skin that can be excised (see Fig 7–1,D). If the amount of skin seems inadequate, further undermining can be undertaken at this point. If more or less skin than initially was planned can be excised, adjustment is made in the location of the second incision.

The second half of the ellipse then is cut and the scalp ellipse removed. Hemostasis on this side of the incision is carried out in the same way, and the wound is ready for closing. We have been extremely gratified with the use of towel clips for this portion of the procedure. The clips are placed along the suture line, holding the entire gaping wound together (Fig 7–1,E). The galeal closure then is easily undertaken without a great deal of tugging and, consequently, less tearing. The clips are removed as we suture our way toward each one (Fig 7–1,F). We cannot emphasize enough how important the use of towel clips is at this stage. The stretching of the scalp with the clips also stretches the dermal collagen so the scalp gradually relaxes over the first five to ten minutes of stretching. This also makes the closure much easier.

The galea is first closed with 1-0 or 2-0 Vicryl on a UR-6 or Dexon on a C-6 needle. We have found that the best results are obtained by using thick buried sutures on half round needles. We routinely use a running suture; however, interrupted buried sutures are acceptable. The skin is closed as a separate layer, using staples or 0 to 000 silk or 3-0 Mersilene, depending on the amount of tension across the wound.

A dressing is optional. Most patients do not require any dressing, but those who feel insecure can have a head wrap for 12–24 hours. The staples or sutures are removed in 10–14 days.

There are two techniques to increase the amount of tissue that can be removed or to close the wound if it is under excessive tension. First, galeotomies can be performed (Fig 7–1,G). These are incisions parallel to the skin incision made through the galea and approximately 1.0 cm apart. To be successful, the galea must be filleted through its entire thickness so that some fat protrudes. At the same time, it is important to incise only the galea because of the deep dermal vessels that sometimes lie just beneath it. These linear incisions may be made with a #15 Bard-Parker blade, with a 75-S Beaver blade or with neurosurgical dura blades that have a cutting end that is only 2.0 mm long. Some surgeons even wrap 1.0 mm of this 2.0-mm cutting edge so that only 1.0 mm of knife is exposed. This makes incisions controllable to a 1.0-mm depth. The galea incisions are made on both sides of the midline as far as the surgeon can conveniently reach and see and preferably in the hair-bearing scalp so that hairy scalp is stretched rather than bald scalp. If a vessel is cut while performing the galeotomies, the surgeon must be able to coagulate or suture it. Often, an additional 1.0 to 2.0 cm of scalp can be excised by the use of multiple galeotomies.

If for some reason the central wound still will not close, relaxing incisions can be made above one or both of the ears. This incision is made in the hair above one or both of the ears with a full cut through the skin, subcutaneous tissue, and galea. Hemostasis is obtained in the usual way and only the skin of this relaxing incision is sutured together. This allows a 0.5–1.0-cm galeal spreading (a percutaneous galeotomy), which then relaxes the central incision. This type of closure should not be part of the surgical planning but used only in those cases in which the central incision cannot be closed primarily. A series of clinical photographs showing our technique is included (see Fig 7–2).

Approximately 50% of the patients believe that scalp reduction was a painful experience. Those who have had hair transplants by the standard method often believe the scalp reduction pain is more enduring. Patients complain of

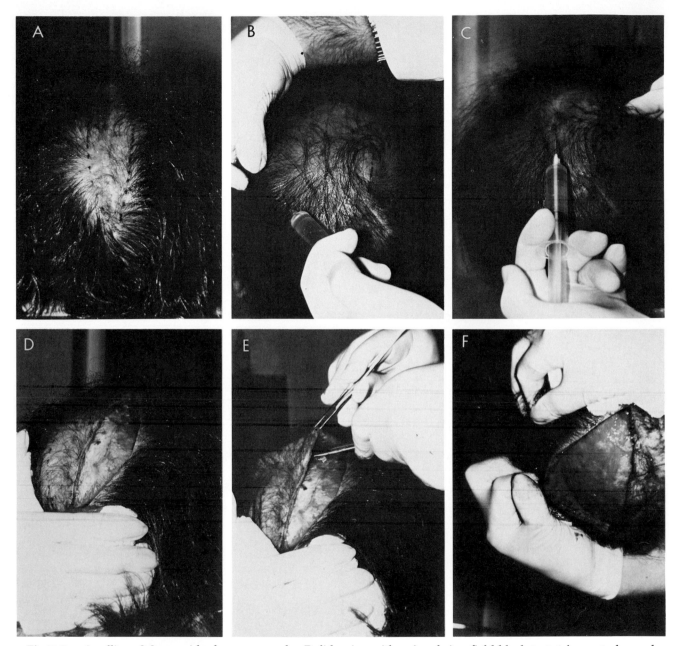

Fig 7–2.—**A,** ellipse 3.0-cm wide drawn on scalp. **B,** lidocaine with epinephrine field block to total area to be undermined. **C,** lidocaine with epinephrine into incision sites for better anesthesia and hemostasis. **D,** one side of ellipse incised. **E,** wide undermining on each side. **F,** checking for bleeders using hair to lift flap. *(continued)*

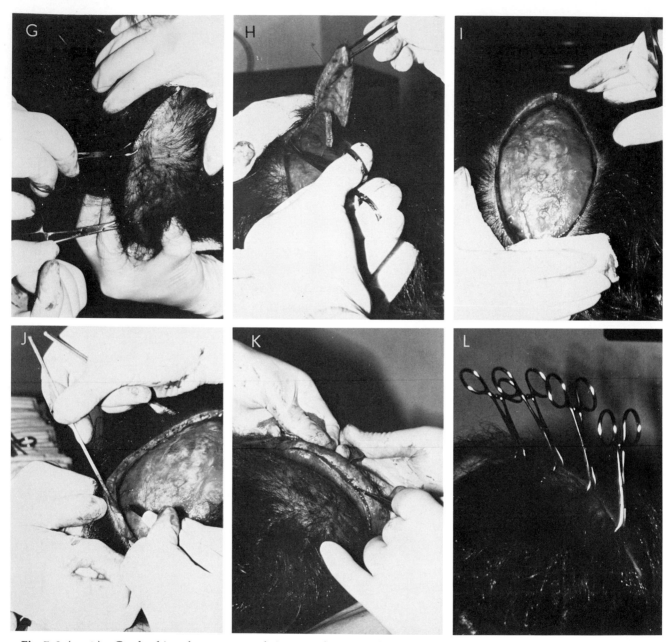

Fig 7–2 (cont.)—G, checking for amount of tissue to be excised. **H,** removing ellipse. Note transverse incision to facilitate removal. **I,** bald scalp excised. **J,** final hemostasis of wound edges. **K,** galeotomies for easier wound closure. **L,** towel clips to take up tension.

pain when sleeping or when trying to eat or smile. Postoperatively, we ordinarily give Tylenol with codeine, Percocet, or combine one of these with Motrin. Some patients need this analgesia only the first 48 hours but others take it for up to ten days.

Hematoma has been the only major complication, and that has been present in less than 1% of the patients. Management of the hematoma is in the stan-

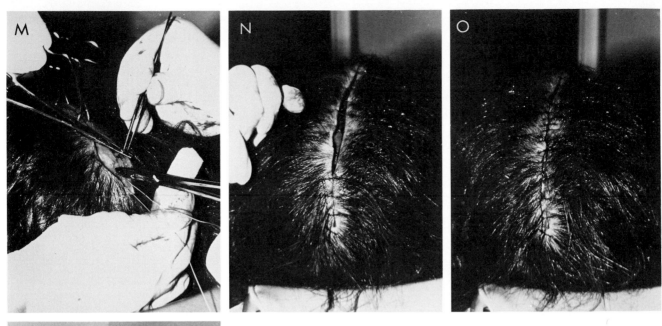

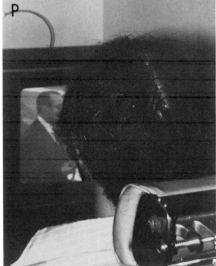

Fig 7–2 (cont.)—**M**, closing galea with running suture. **N**, closing skin with running locked suture. **O**, closure almost completed. **P**, patient stays in chair he has been in during procedure in order to finish viewing TV program.

dard fashion by releasing a few of the stitches, expressing the clot, and obtaining hemostasis. The subgaleal plane then is irrigated with sterile normal saline and the wound closed. It has become our practice to suture approximately 5.0–10.0 mm beyond the distal ends of the incision line. This places a percutaneous suture through the galea and catches some bleeders that may be present at either end of the suture line but are not caught up in the buried running stitch.

Occasionally there has been some inversion of the scar line, but this has been minimized greatly since we have been routinely performing the closure of the galea. Hypertrophic scars and keloids could be expected. However, we have not encountered them to date. A few patients had thin, spread scars. Many patients have had scalp reductions who had previous hair transplants, and undermining below these transplants does not seem to disturb the transplants. If hair transplants are performed or existing before scalp reduction, in the presurgical planning the surgeon should remember that the lateral edges of the frontal hairline will be moved in a medial direction depending on the amount of scalp removed at that level of the anterior crown. This is important if there is much built-in recession of the frontal hairline. In some cases, if several scalp reductions will be done, frontal hair plugs are put in a straight line before scalp reduction. Sometimes additional plugs in the frontal line become necessary.

If there is a significant loss of hair in the posterior portion of the crown, an

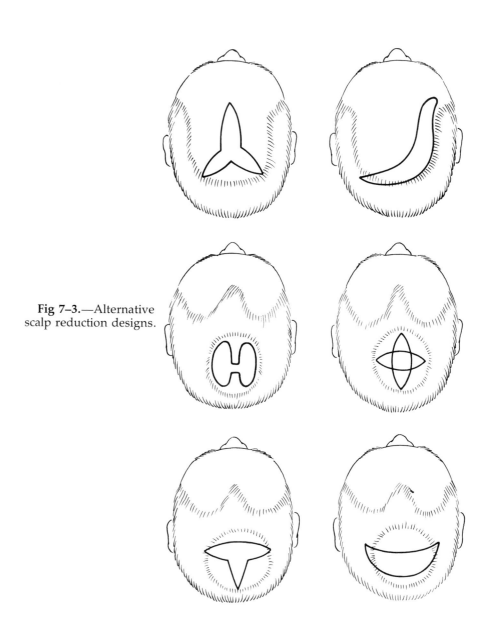

Fig 7–3.—Alternative scalp reduction designs.

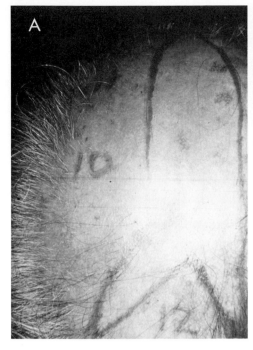

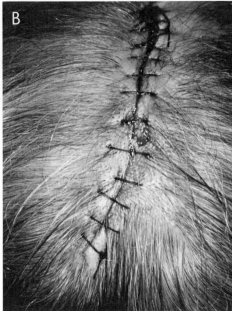

Fig 7–4.—A, before scalp reduction.
B, after fourth scalp reduction.

M-plasty (Fig 7–3) at the posterior end of the elliptical incision has become our favorite form of management. This design eliminates not only scalp in a side-to-side manner but also a great deal of the crown baldness. Two clinical cases are shown (Figs 7–4 and 7–5). This technique is immensely successful, but has

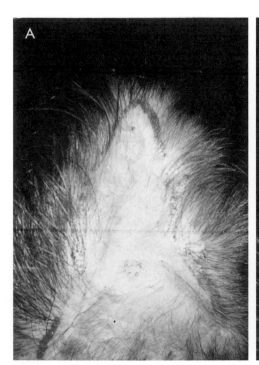

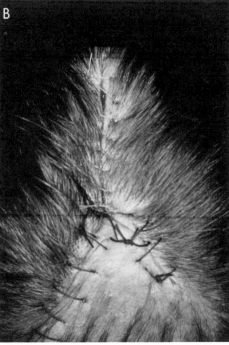

Fig 7–5.—A, before scalp reduction.
B, after scalp reduction.

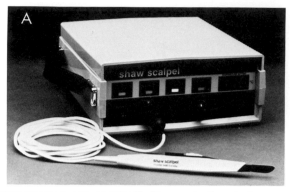

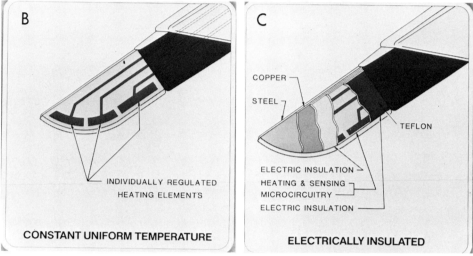

Fig 7–6.—Shaw scalpel, electronic scalpel that seals bleeders as it cuts, using direct heat **(A to C).**

the one design drawback: a flap tip is created. Where these tips converge there is a concentration of suture material. With the thick sutures that are used for the galea, this often can lead to an inflammatory response and even to tip necrosis. Usually, tip necrosis or inflammation eventually heals without any difficulty or obvious scarring. It is a temporary complication.

It is our preference to perform the simple ellipse or the ellipse with the M-plasty in the crown and then repeat the procedure as needed rather than to do some of the larger, more complicated procedures. We believe that the 2.0–3.0 cm greater width of scalp that can be removed is not merited by the increased operative morbidity and cost. Since a repeated scalp reduction can be performed as soon as six weeks later, we believe it is wiser to do two or three scalp reductions that are simple and relatively less traumatic than to do one very large one. This philosophy varies among surgeons. More scalp could be removed if a three- to six-month waiting period between reductions were allowed. However, patients often are anxious to complete the entire procedure in the shortest time possible, so we ask them to wait the six to twelve weeks before their second reduction. Sometimes transplants can be placed along the frontal hairline or along the parietal edges of the scalp before a second reduction is undertaken. Try to harvest transplants from the sides of the scalp above the ears and in the posterior lateral portion of the hair-bearing scalp before several scalp reductions stretch this part of the scalp and reduce the density of the hair.

There are several other patterns for scalp reductions. The J-shaped or S-shaped paramedian incision (see Fig 7–3) is popular and has been well described by Thomas Alt.[5] With this method, which can be done on both sides of the scalp, there are no tips of flaps that may easily necrose. This crescentic wound is partially closed with side-to-side movement and with some rotation of the scalp that facilitates its movement and allows a larger amount of tissue to be removed.

If the baldness is only in the crown, the butterfly-shaped reduction or the star-shaped reduction (see Fig 7–3) is applicable. Depending on the shape of the skull, a T-shaped excision or C-shaped excision (see Fig 7–3) also is a good way to reduce the skin from the posterior crown.

Recently we had the opportunity to do scalp reduction with the Shaw scalpel (Fig 7–6). This electronic device uses #15- or #10-sized blades. The blade is coated with copper and Teflon except for the cutting edge. Microcircuits beneath the Teflon layer maintain the cutting edge at temperatures of 110 F to 260 F, which can be selected by a button on the handle. A bar switch on the handle raises the blade temperatures rapidly to 270 F for instant hemostasis of larger vessels. This blade seals small vessels by direct thermal heat as it cuts and greatly speeds the scalp reduction. With continued favorable experience this has certainly become our favorite tool for the incision in scalp reduction.

CONCLUSION

Scalp reduction now is an integral part of hair transplantation when done by either the Orentreich method or the flap method. At the initial consultation, the whole process, i.e., hair redistribution by plug or flap and scalp reduction, is planned. If a patient is to have hair plugs and scalp reduction, the hairline usually is put in first because of the three-month waiting time for the hair to begin to grow. We do the first scalp reduction a month later and continue with scalp reductions until hair from the plugs is sufficiently long to facilitate the placing of filler grafts in the front line and the rows behind. Since the scalp reduction will raise the hairline, particularly at the recessions, this movement of hairline is programmed into the plan so that the hair plugs at the side are placed slightly lower than when scalp reduction is not done. Similarly, if a combination flap and scalp reduction(s) is planned, the flap(s) is done first and scalp reduction started a month or more later.

REFERENCES

1. Blanchard G., Blanchard B.: Obliteration of alopecia by hair-lifting: a new concept and technique. *J. Natl. Med. Assoc.* 69:639–641, 1977.
2. Blanchard G., Blanchard B.: La réduction tonsurale (détonsuration): Concept nouveau dans le traitement chirurgical de la calvitie. *Rev. Chir. Esth. L. Fr.* 4:5–10, 1976.
3. Stough D.B., Webster R.C.: *Esthetics and Refinements in Hair Transplantation.* Lucerne, Switzerland, The International Hair Transplant Symposium, Feb. 4, 1978.

4. Sparkuhl K.: *Scalp Reduction: Serial Excision of the Scalp with Flap Advancement.* Lucerne, Switzerland, The International Hair Transplant Symposium, Feb. 4, 1978.
5. Alt T.: Scalp reduction. *Cosmet. Surg.* 1:1–19, 1981.
6. Unger M.G., Unger W.P.: Management of alopecia of the scalp by a combination of excision and transplantations. *J. Dermatol. Surg. Oncol.* 4:670–672, 1978.
7. Bosley L.L., Hope C.R., Montroy R.E.: Male pattern reduction (MPR)™ for surgical reduction of male pattern baldness. *Curr. Ther. Res.* 25:281–287, 1979.
8. Schultz B.D., Roenigk H.H. Jr.: Scalp reduction for alopecia. *J. Dermatol. Surg. Oncol.* 5:808–811, 1979.
9. Bosley L.L., Hope C.R., Montroy R.E.: Scalp reduction for alopecia. *J. Dermatol. Surg. Oncol.* 6:498, 503, 1980.
10. Bell M.L.: The role of scalp reduction in the treatment of male pattern alopecia. *Plast. Reconstr. Surg.* 69:272–277, 1982.

8 / Scalp Flaps for Alopecia

FLAPS PROBABLY will be used much less often than scalp reduction or hair transplants for the management of male pattern alopecia, but they are an important adjunct to the armamentarium. They can be used in conjunction with scalp reduction and transplants, and for some people may be the only surgical treatment necessary. Jose Juri published his work on the use of the parieto-occipital flaps in 1975.[1] This bold and masterful flap was the innovation needed to demonstrate that flaps could be an important method of covering alopecia. Since that time there have been several modifications of the flap, as well as further papers by the Juri brothers and others,[2–6] all of which demonstrate that this flap and its variations are practical and lasting methods.

OUR PREFERRED FLAP

The flap that we have come to use most commonly is a modification of the Lamont flap, which originally was described in 1957 and later published by D. Bluford Stough.[7, 8] The Stough modification involves one delay and also narrows the proximal end of the flap so that the problem with the rotation dog-ear is minimized. Also, designing the flap around a proved location of the central branch of the temporal artery has become less important, and, therefore, the flap can be designed more to meet the patient's hair pattern and to obviate the formation of a large rotation dog-ear. These modifications have made the flap more simple; thus it is amenable to office cosmetic surgery. We have performed this flap with the patient sitting up in a barber-type chair, but believe that for most patients it should be done in the office surgery with the patient supine and with the support of IV fluids and medications.

The indications for a large flap are patients with alopecia limited to the frontal one-third to one-half of the scalp; women who have a temporal recession and need to have a rounder, more feminine hairline; and patients with extensive alopecia in whom there are not adequate donor sites for punch transplants. For the last indication, one or two of the large flaps, followed by scalp reduction, will give the patient a full-appearing frontal hairline and the ability to let the hair grow long and comb over the remaining balding portions at the posterior parts of the scalp. Another indication is patients who do not want the irregular plugged effect of frontal hairline after the usual punch transplants.

The procedure is much more difficult for the patient and the physician than either scalp reduction or punch transplants. The results are immediate. Most patients are gratified and believe that the procedure and costs were well justified.

TECHNIQUE

The modification of the flap that we now perform most often starts by designing a flap that has its origin at approximately a 40-degree angle to the horizontal plane 1.0–2.0 cm anterior to the leading edge of the pinna and 1.0–2.0 cm superior to the anterior edge of the insertion of the helix. Although the temporal artery or branches of the temporal artery may be palpated or identified with a Doppler apparatus, this probably is unnecessary, since the entire blood supply of this area is rich with the temporal artery supply and the flap does not need to be designed with a branch of that artery in the center of the flap. The anatomy of this artery and its branches varies greatly, and rigid adherence to a design that calls for an artery within the flap would alter the design of the flap from patient to patient. The width of the flap at the rotation point is between 2.5 and 2.8 cm. The original flaps were 3.0–4.0 cm in width throughout their length. Stough and others have shown that the proximal end of the flap does not need to be as wide as the distal end, and this narrowing has been one of the major factors in reducing the bulkiness of the rotation dog-ear. The flap is designed as a gentle *S* that extends over the parietal area and around the edge of the lambdoid ridge, not quite to the midline of the posterior scalp. The flap can be any length shorter if the patient has high, hair-bearing sides of the scalp. It should be full length for a patient with a wide scalp who will require a flap from both sides to complete the frontal hairline. The flap distal to the rotation point is quickly widened to 3.0 cm and terminates posteriorly in a 30-degree angle to facilitate closure in the occipital area.

Various techniques are used to map out the flap. Some surgeons use a simple school compass with marking pens attached to the ends so that the width of the flap can be drawn evenly. Others create a tape or foam rubber template of the entire flap, lay it over the scalp, and trace around the edge with marking pens. Both of these methods are quite helpful in the original design. A rat-toothed comb facilitates separating the hair on the flap from the hair on the remaining scalp. The hair on the flap is pulled together with bobby pins or rubber bands and kept out of the way of the surgical incision. Next, the frontal hairline should be drawn. It need not be a simple curve, but can be S-shaped, which is more natural. Definite temporal recessions should be drawn. The patient should participate in the location and drawing of the frontal hairline. Then some sort of a malleable template should be used to rotate as the flap will rotate, to estimate roughly how much of the frontal hairline can be achieved or how long the flap should be. Estimates are somewhat unpredictable, since the amount of rotation dog-ear formed varies if the side of the scalp easily moves superiorly. The more the base moves, the more the flap will cover the frontal hairline. There also is a surprising amount of extensibility of the flap as it is sutured into place.

Using 1% Xylocaine with epinephrine as anesthesia, the first delay is accomplished. The skin is incised through the level of the galea for the posterior one-half of the flap (Fig 8–1,A). Hemostasis is obtained with electrodesiccation or suture ligatures as needed. Some surgeons undermine this area of the scalp at this time to lessen bleeding when the flap is later transferred. The posterior one-half of the flap then is lifted all the way from the scalp bed and replaced.

The skin is sewed side to side with the suture material of choice, we use 3-0 Mersilene suture. A head wrap is placed for 24 hours and the patient's activities are limited. This delay should be performed 10–20 days before the full flap procedure. The delay theoretically increases the blood supply to the flap through the narrow pedicle by forcing the blood supply to come through that pedicle. Whether this is a neovascularization, a hypertrophy of the existing vessels, or has to do with the relaxation of the autonomic nervous system's influence over the arterial vessels is subject to speculation.

On the day of the next surgery, the entire scalp is cleansed. Some surgeons prefer a Betadine scrub of the scalp and lateral neck down to the level of the shoulders; others have their patients shampoo the morning of surgery or use Hibiclens in the shower before coming to the office. The patients should have an IV started with D5W and 0.5 normal saline solution, and it is helpful to monitor cardiac status and blood pressure. The flap is redrawn as it originally was drawn and the hair near the incision site is tied out of the way. Local anesthesia is achieved with Xylocaine with epinephrine 1:100,000. It should extend well down onto the neck in all areas that will be undermined.

The flap is cut along its entirety and elevated (Fig 8–1,B). Hemostasis is obtained with electrodesiccation and suture ligatures. Some surgeons prefer to use hot cautery or suture ligatures on the flap itself to avoid electrodesiccation which may extend along the path of the artery and compromise more of the artery than is necessary. Undermining is started along the entire length of the flap and extends to the level of the pinna. The undermining may extend onto the posterior aspect of the pinna and onto the neck. This undermining should be done under direct visualization; therefore, a head lamp or good ceiling lighting is necessary. One or two assistants and long instruments of the type used in thoracic or abdominal surgery also are needed.

Once this entire area is undermined, the proposed anterior hairline is incised. This incision is made with a bevel starting posteriorly and aiming anteriorly (Fig 8–1,C). This bevel will match with a trimming of the leading edge of the flap. Some of the hairs on the leading edge of the flap are trimmed just above the base of the hair papillae. These hairs will grow through the scar, camouflaging the scar and making the frontal hairline appear more natural. This technique originally was described to his students by Juri but was first published in the United States by Sheldon Kabaker. It is extremely effective in camouflaging this otherwise obvious hairline scar.[4, 5]

Once the anterior hairline is incised, the central portion of the scalp is undermined in the subgaleal plane, and the donor area is closed side to side. Dexon 1-0 on a C-6 needle is our suture of choice. We make a deep bite through the galea and come up into the middermal region with large interrupted sutures. This is the most difficult and critical portion of the surgery, but once it is completed, the remainder of surgery, although time-consuming, is without anxiety. If the donor site should fail to close, more undermining can be undertaken. Relaxing incisions can be made in the parietal scalp or actually up on the central scalp if necessary. These relaxing incisions are essentially full-thickness cuts through the skin and galea with resuturing of the skin only. The resulting gap in the galea gives 1.0 cm more of closing ability. If the donor areas still cannot be closed, some of the bald scalp that will be excised in the recipient area to allow for the flap can be used as a temporary full-thickness

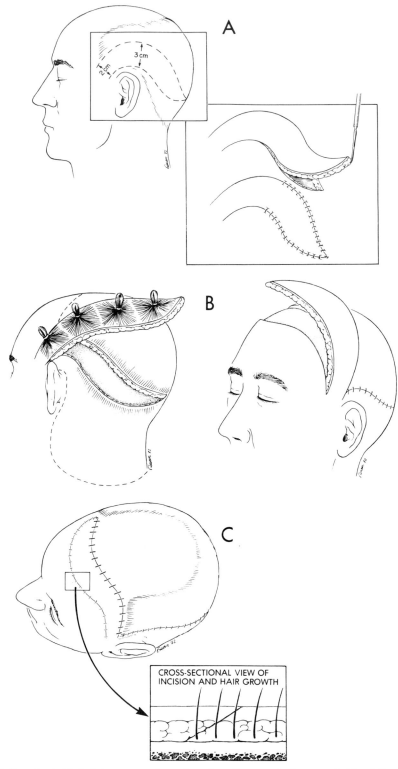

Fig 8–1.—A, initial delay procedure by elevating posterior one-half of flap. **B,** the whole flap is incised. **C,** an anteriorly beveled incision is made and the flap transposed into place.

graft in the donor area until the entire scalp shifts and stretches. Some months later, this graft can be excised and the area closed primarily.

With the donor site closed, the flap is carefully laid into the defect created by the incision of the anterior hairline. Try not to pull on the flap or put it under tension in either direction. If a large dog-ear results, the adjacent forehead and temple should be widely undermined. Suturing starts at the proximal end of the flap on its leading edge. Fine 5-0 or 6-0 Prolene, nylon, or Ethiflex sutures are preferable. Meticulous interrupted sutures gradually approximate the scalp to the forehead, and, as this is done, the flap can be nudged gently forward. It will stretch a fair amount. With this technique and forehead undermining, the dog-ear is minimized. Once the anterior edge of the flap is sutured, an appropriate amount of bald scalp is excised and discarded. Staples can be used for the posterior edge of the flap and the closure of the donor site. If there is a large discrepancy between the thickness of the flap and the thickness of the scalp along the posterior edge of the flap, vertical mattress sutures may be needed to approximate this area, and then staples can be used between these mattress sutures.

If there is a great deal of oozing, a drain can be left in place, usually about the area of the rotation dog-ear. The patient then should be observed for 30–60 minutes. Our patients are given a head wrap and sent home with oral analgesics consisting of Tylenol with codeine, Percocet, Motrin, or a combination of these.

The postoperative morbidity, as might be expected, involves swelling of the forehead and ecchymoses on the posterior scalp, the neck, postauricular area, the forehead, and around the eyes. These are common sequelae, but whether the use of corticosteroids at the time of surgery or just after is helpful has yet to be scientifically determined. We routinely give our patients prophylactic antibiotics.

Stitches and staples are removed between seven and 14 days as indicated. Sometimes there is loss of some of the hair at the distal end of the flap. Most of the time, this hair will regrow in two to three months. Sometimes there is necrosis of the tip of the flap, but this can be repaired by excision and primary closure or repaired when a second flap is done from the opposite side. Occasionally, a telogen effluvium occurs at the donor site.

There are various techniques for using two flaps. Some are placed side to side, making the frontal area up to 6.0 cm thick, and then the rest of the scalp is treated with scalp reduction or transplants. Sometimes a second flap is placed 2.0–3.0 cm behind the first flap and the intervening bald area is reduced later in the standard scalp reduction fashion.

It is our belief that this flap modification will become the most popular one because of its decreased morbidity and complications and, therefore, results in less cost and risk to the patient (Figs 8–2 and 8–3). The quite large flap, as originally described by Juri, always will remain in use, but is for those patients who can afford the time and money for the double delay and the morbidity of the extensive surgery to have a 4.0-cm-wide hairline with one flap.

The advantages of the flap are that the hair replacement is instant and there is no need for three long months of waiting for the hair to grow. With modifications by trimming the anterior edge of the flap, the frontal hairline has become more and more normal-appearing. Fleming and Mayer in Los Angeles

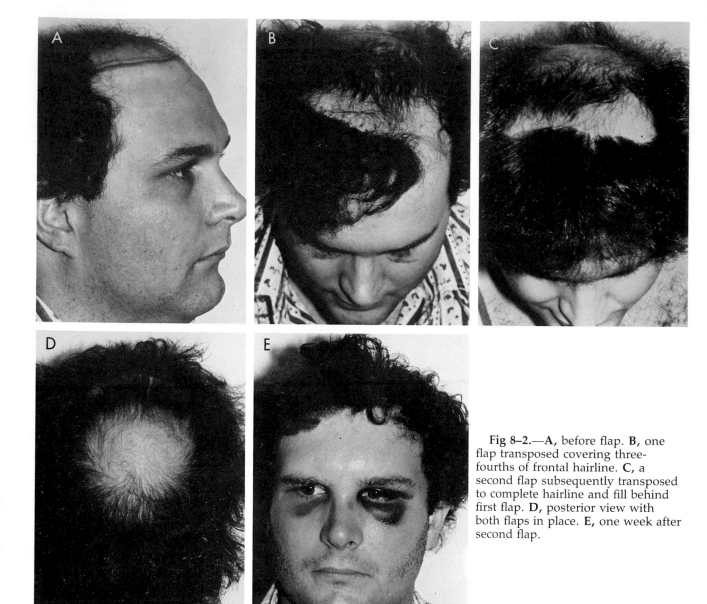

Fig 8–2.—A, before flap. **B,** one flap transposed covering three-fourths of frontal hairline. **C,** a second flap subsequently transposed to complete hairline and fill behind first flap. **D,** posterior view with both flaps in place. **E,** one week after second flap.

encouraged the shaping of the frontal hairline into an S-shaped pattern, which is easily done at the time of the surgery and greatly reduces the sharp artificial appearance of some of the earlier Juri-type flaps.[3]

The disadvantages of hair flaps are that the hair grows straight back, and some effort must be made to style and tease the hair to one side or the other. A "whorl" develops at the site of the rotation of the flap, and this requires camouflaging with hairstyling. The surgeon should be hesitant to do a large flap if the patient would be unhappy needing to camouflage this rotation whorl and to have to comb the hair in a specific direction.

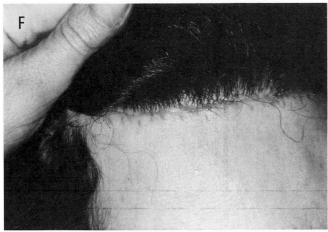

Fig 8–2. (cont.)—F, close-up of hairline showing some hairs growing through scar tissue. **G,** six months after last flap.

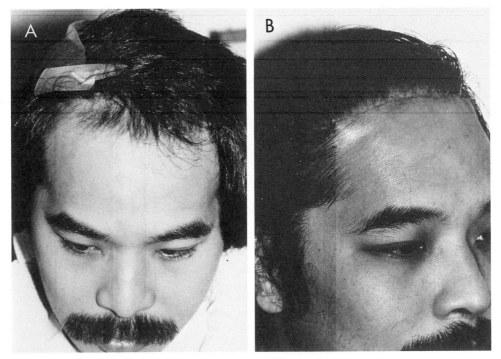

Fig 8–3.—A, before flaps. **B,** two flaps done. Hair combed backward to show linear scar.

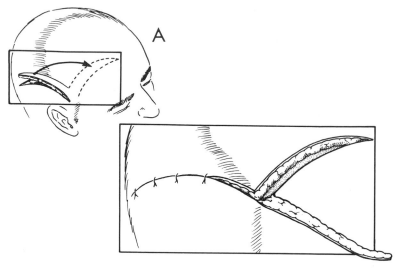

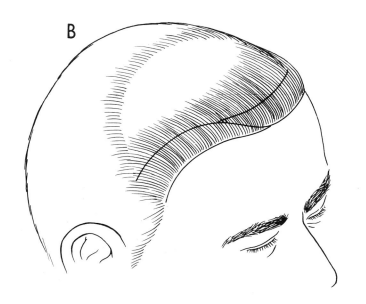

Fig 8–4.—A, short temporal flap. *Left,* flap elevated; *right,* donor site closed and flap being transposed into frontal hairline. **B,** two short temporal flaps interconnecting at midline.

SHORT TEMPORAL FLAPS

In the American literature in 1957 Lamont described a technique of constructing short, bilateral and roughly symmetric flaps overlapping in the mid-frontal portion of the scalp to provide an anterior hairline.[9] These flaps did not require any delay. A flap from one side was turned to provide half of the hairline. After a month or more, to be sure that the first flap was well healed, a second flap would be turned from the other side to complete the hairline. These 2.0- to 3.0-cm wide flaps could be turned and the donor sites closed primarily. Passot in 1931 had described a similar procedure, and Heimburger in 1977 again rediscovered the technique some 20 years after the paper by Lamont.[10, 11] However, it was Elliott, Jr., who did a series of these flaps to explore the benefits and possible side effects in many patients.[12] He demonstrated that these short flaps provided instant hair since the hairs did not go into telogen, resulting in loss of hair. Rarely, some hair was lost at the tip of the flap, but almost all of the hair continued to grow.

The flaps are generally 2.0 cm wide although 2.5-cm-wide flaps can be used (Fig 8–4,A). The base of the flap is designed so that the full force of the branches of the superficial temporal artery will nourish the flap. The length of the flap is determined by the distance from the base of the flap to the midline of the proposed hairline adding to this figure a 25%–40% increase in flap length (Fig 8–4,B). This additional flap length is lost in turning the flap into place with the creation of a dog-ear. It is better to err on the long side, since extra flap length can always be extended across the frontal hairline toward the other side. Then a shorter flap would be needed at the second procedure. The cutting of the flaps, undermining, hemostasis, and closure is the same as described above.

The advantage of the short, temporal 2.0-cm flaps is that they can be done in one sitting, and since each flap is nourished by a different artery, the second flap can be done with only a month's delay between procedures. Both flaps could actually be done at the same session. The 2.0-cm-wide flaps provide a frontal hairline with enough hair to give a dense look. Plugs and other flaps can be placed behind them. Again, the hair is growing in a posterior direction instead of the normal forward direction, but the dense frontal hairline is preferable to many people. The instant hair obtained outweighs the negative fea-

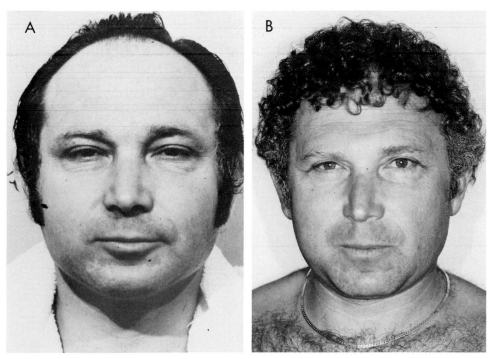

Fig 8–5.—**A,** before short temporal flaps. **B,** following two short temporal flaps and hair permanent. (Courtesy of Drs. Toby Mayer and Richard Fleming, Beverly Hills, Calif.)

ture of the direction of the hair growth. The biggest negative feature is that the short temporal flaps blunt the temporal recessions. The inability to make sufficient temporal recessions and the hair's growing in the wrong direction result in significantly poorer cosmetic results than can be obtained with the longer flaps. Whether to do these short flaps, the 3.0-cm long flap described above, or the 4.0-cm Juri flap depends on the individual patient and physician.

With each of these flaps, the best candidates are patients with curly, kinky, or wavy hair so the effect of the hair growing backward instead of in the normal forward direction will be disguised or muted. Probably the worst candidates are patients with straight, wiry hair with large shafts that accentuate the fact that hair is growing backward instead of forward. The ideal candidates are those who plan to permanent wave their hair or always style their hair so not only is the hair growth direction disguised but also the frontal hairline and the whorl from the dog-ear is hidden (Fig 8–5).

REFERENCES

1. Juri J.: Use of parieto-occipital flaps in the surgical treatment of baldness. *Plast. Reconstr. Surg.* 55:456–460, 1975.
2. Juri J.: Use of rotation scalp flaps for treatment of occipital baldness. *Plast. Reconstr. Surg.* 61:23–26, 1978.
3. Mayer T.G., Flemming R.W.: Short versus long scalp flaps in the treatment of male pattern baldness. *Arch. Otolaryngol.* 107:403–408, 1981.
4. Kabaker S.: Experiences with parieto-occipital flaps in hair transplantation. *Laryngoscope* 88:73–84, 1978.
5. Kabaker S.: Juri flap procedure for the treatment of baldness. *Arch. Otolaryngol.* 105:509–514, 1979.
6. Rabineau P.: Surgical treatment of baldness using Juri's technique. *Cutis* 25:511–515, 1980.
7. Stough III D.B., Cates J.A.: Transposition flaps for the correction of baldness: a practical office procedure. *J. Dermatol. Surg. Oncol.* 6:286–289, 1980.
8. Stough III D.B., Cates J.A., Dean A.J.: Updating reduction and flap procedures for baldness. *Ann. Plast. Surg.* 8:287–295, 1982.
9. Lamont E.S.: A plastic surgical transformation. *West. J. Surg. Gynecol.* 65:164–165, 1957.
10. Passot R.: *Chirurgie Esthetique Pure Technique et Resultats.* Paris, Doin & Cie, 1931.
11. Heimburger R.A.: Single stage rotation of arterialized scalp flaps for male pattern baldness: case report. *Plast. Reconstr. Surg.* 60:789–790, 1977.
12. Elliott R.A., Jr.: Lateral scalp flaps for instant results in male pattern baldness. *Plast. Reconstr. Surg.* 60:699–703, 1977.

9 / Injectable Collagen

IN THE EARLY 1970s, four investigators at Stanford University were working on different potential uses for collagen. Rodney Perkins of Otolaryngology, John Daniels in Internal Medicine and Biochemistry, Edward Lock, a medical student, and Terrence Knapp in Plastic Surgery then combined forces to focus on development of a clinically useful collagen material.[1, 2] This material, an injectable collagen implant with the trade name Zyderm, has shown promising results for the correction of soft depressed contour deformities and early wrinkles and creases. The manufacturer, Collagen Corporation (Palo Alto, Calif.), received marketing approval from the FDA in August 1981.

Collagen is one of the least toxic and least irritating biomaterials known. In the manufacture of this product, bovine dermis is solubilized in a nondestructive fashion through selective hydrolysis of the telopeptide end regions of the collagen molecule. This hydrolysis leads to a reduction of the intermolecular and intramolecular cross-links while preserving the integrity of the main body of the collagen molecule. It is believed that this process further reduces the already very low antigenetic potential of this material. It then is sterilized and purified by process conditions that lead to a sterile, pyrogen-free product. This manufacturing process differentiates Zyderm collagen from other currently used medical collagen products such as hemostatic agents, blood vessel prostheses, and sutures that are derived either directly from biologic membranes or from dispersions of collagen fibers.

Zyderm collagen is packaged in a sterile syringe, 0.1 ml for skin testing and 0.5, 1.0, and 2.0 ml for implantation. It is stored at -4 C (refrigerator temperature) to reduce the tendency of the molecules to reform into fibers while still in the syringe. When the material is brought to homeostatic conditions at 37.5 C, 7.4 pH, etc., on its implantation it undergoes a fibrous transformation that changes it from an opalescent gel suspension to an opaque semisolid. For this reason, it should be kept refrigerated or in a cool ice carrier until just before its injection. As the material now is distributed to the physician, the gel contains 30%–35% or 65% bovine collagen by wet weight, suspended in a buffered physiologic saline solution containing 0.3% lidocaine. The 35% is called Zyderm I and the 65% Zyderm II.

Extensive animal studies were done in rats that showed that when the material was injected into the subcutaneous tissue, an early inflammatory cell infiltrate developed that was sparse and transient. Macroscopically, the implant appeared cohesive, uniform, and vascularized on its surface, with no attempts by the host to wall off the implant or form a thick, fibrous capsule. Microscopically, the implant showed colonization over a 90-day period by host fibroblasts and evidence of neovascularization through the implant.

The histologic appearance of the implant in humans is different from that of

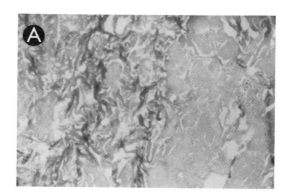

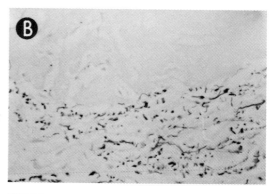

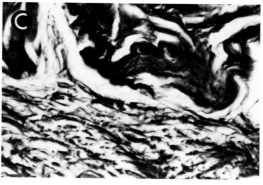

Fig 9–1.—Four months postinjection of implanted Zyderm collagen. **A,** hematoxylin-eosin stain; × 80. **B,** Verhoeff's elastic stain reveals no elastic staining fibers growing into the implant and no evidence of capsular formation around the implant; × 80. **C,** stained with colloidal iron and counterstained with acid fuchsin. Shows the bright purple color *(top)* of the implant vs. the red-pink color *(bottom)* of the native collagen; × 80.

the rat model. Early data supplied by the manufacturer indicate that the contour correction subsides only 20%–30% in the first 12–14 months.[3] Two hypotheses might explain the difference between human and animal experience. In humans, Zyderm implant is placed into the dermis, where it is completely surrounded by native collagen rather than the subcutaneous tissues, where it was placed in rats. Second, there would be a difference in the stress on the implant within the collagen of human wrinkles or depressed scars as opposed to simply lying in the subcutaneous area of the rat model.

Biopsy specimens of human implants at four months postinjection show the implanted collagen bundles clearly with the hematoxylin-eosin stain (Fig 9–1,A). The Zyderm implant stains lighter than the normal collagen bundles and shows thicker, more amorphous bundles than in the native collagen. There is no evidence of degradation of the implant and no giant cells or granuloma formation is evident. The elastic stain reveals no elastic staining fibrils growing into the implant but, more importantly, neither is there capsular formation around the implant (Fig 9–1,B). There is a distinct tinctorial difference from normal collagen when observed by the colloidal iron stain that has been counterstained with acid fuchsin (Fig 9–1,C). The Zyderm collagen stains a bright violet-purple as opposed to the red-pinkish color of the native collagen. Also, with the colloidal iron stain there is no evidence of glucoseaminoglycans or excess new collagen formation by the host around the implant. Zyderm collagen also can be differentiated by trichrome stain.

Biopsy specimens taken of positive skin tests—that is, collagen skin tests that were clinically determined to be positive because of induration, pruritus, or persistent or exaggerated erythema—show invasion of the collagen implant fibers by host monocytes (Fig 9–2,A). These cellular responses range from monocyte-only infiltrates to mixed cellular infiltrates with eosinophils, polymorphonuclear leukocytes, and foreign-body giant cells (Figs 9–2,B and C).

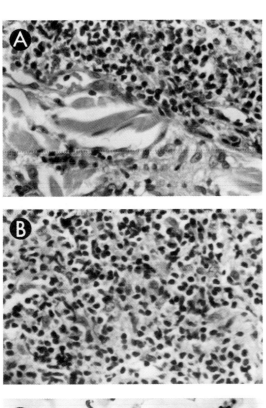

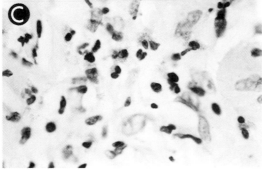

Fig 9–2.—Biopsy specimen of a positive skin test. **A & B,** stained with hematoxylin-eosin; × 200. Showing massive infiltrate of eosinophiles, polymorphonuclear leukocytes, and foreign body giant cells. **C,** stained with hematoxylin-eosin; × 1,000. Shows the reaction with a predominance of eosinophiles.

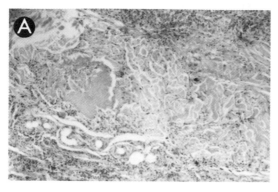
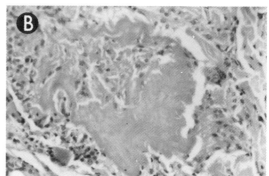
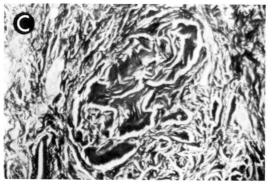

Fig 9–3.—A, biopsy specimen taken from acquired allergy to Zyderm collagen implant (patient had negative skin test). Showing a foreign-body type reaction. Hematoxylin-eosin stain; × 24. B, same as above; × 80. C, stained with colloidal iron; × 24.

Biopsy specimens from persons with acquired allergies to Zyderm (patients whose skin tests were negative and later had induration and erythema at the treatment sites—usually with a similar response at the formerly negative skin test site) showed a similar foreign-body type reaction (Figs 9–3,A and B). To date these reactions at treatment sites have had fewer polymorphonuclear leukocytes and more monocytes and giant cells. On the low-power views of the hematoxylin-eosin stain, it is easy to see how one could confuse this reaction with any reaction that involves a necrobiotic collagen. The surrounding and invading monocytes with the amorphous center collagen material appear very much like granuloma annulare, rheumatoid nodules, foreign-body reactions, and necrobiosis lipoidica diabeticorum.[4] However, when the same specimens from treatment site reactions are stained with colloidal iron, it is likely that the central collagen material is the Zyderm implant because of the violet-purple distinctive tinctorial difference (Fig 9–3,C).

PATIENT SCREENING

Prospective patients for collagen injection are screened. Those who have a personal history of rheumatic diseases, collagen diseases, or "autoimmune" diseases are arbitrarily excluded. There is no theoretical evidence that bovine collagen injection would cause problems in these patients. Until a greater mass of human data support this conjecture, however, and a controlled study is done in which patients with a history of collagen vascular disease are injected, it is probably prudent to eliminate as candidates these people. Antibodies to the Zyderm implant have been raised in human beings and appear in about

50% of the patients with positive skin test results. These antibodies do not cross-react with human collagen. In some of the patients who have received Zyderm and have developed antibodies to the Zyderm there has been no associated clinical disease or condition.

Collagen vascular diseases seem to develop in patients with certain genetic predispositions as determined by the HLA typing methods plus an inciting event, such as a viral disease, and are limited to certain sex- and age-predetermined patients. No doubt there will be patients who on a chance basis develop these conditions and who have been treated with Zyderm. It will be important that these patients be studied carefully to see whether the Zyderm implant is clinically and histologically involved in whatever collagen vascular disease the patient manifests. Studies at the University of California in San Francisco show that the Zyderm implant is predominantly a type I collagen with trace amounts of type III collagen, whereas lupus erythematosus is associated with a basement membrane antigen, and rheumatoid arthritis is associated with an anti-type II collagen antibody. Dermatomyositis has antibodies directed against muscle tissue. There seems to be little theoretical danger that the use of this implant might lead to one of these so-called collagen vascular diseases. However, at no time should patients be placed at risk.

After an appropriate history has been taken, the prospective patients are given 0.1 ml of Zyderm as a skin test into the volar forearm. The site is evaluated over four weeks to ascertain whether the patient has an allergy to the material. The physician or his staff should observe the skin test site at 48–72 hours. Some patients are so desirous of having the implant that they will "overlook" a positive reaction. Also, some reactions are transient—lasting only 24–48 hours.

Typically, the fluid part of the injection is carried away within a few hours and a small residual amount of collagen remains in the area, but it generally is flat and almost impossible to palpate after a month. Sometimes, if the test site is placed high in the dermis in an area where the volar skin is quite thin, a tiny, yellowish plaque can be observed a month later. A positive test is one with erythema and induration greater than 5.0 mm persisting for several days after injection. To date, approximately 2.5%–3% of the patients tested have shown a positive response to the skin test.[5] Fifty percent of the test reactions occurred within the first 24 hours and over 70% within the first 72 hours, making the first few days important in the test observation. However, some reactions did not occur for more than three weeks following implantation. Consequently, the area should be observed for a full month before being declared negative and before the patient is treated.

INJECTION TECHNIQUES

Our current injection techniques are based on past successes and failures. When we were clinical investigators initially using Zyderm collagen, we found the following procedures *not* helpful: injecting the implant material into the fat to elevate a scar, and injecting around an acne scar. We also tried several scar-releasing techniques, none of which was helpful. These included incising the base of the acne scar deep in the dermis and filling the space with Zyderm collagen, and inserting a hypodermic needle into the skin, cutting the scar with instruments inserted through the needle, and implanting Zyderm collagen in that space. With these techniques, suture closure of the newly created pocket to insure Zyderm collagen placement also was not helpful.

All our injections for Zyderm I are done with a 30-gauge needle. The 27-gauge needle currently supplied by the manufacturer is discarded and a #30 Becton Dickinson plastic hub needle is attached. Only certain brands of 30-gauge needles fit the syringes supplied by Collagen Corporation, and with some brands, the material leaks from the hub. The smaller, 30-gauge needle causes the patient less discomfort on insertion and affords us better control. In thin skin we are better able to maintain the tip of the needle within the dermis. Further, because a 30-gauge needle has a shorter bevel than a 27-gauge needle, there is less chance of placing the bevel partly in the dermis and partly in a pilosebaceous opening with resultant extrusion of Zyderm collagen onto the skin's surface. Also, a bevel partly in dermis and partly in fat would result in most of the Zyderm following the line of least resistance—into the fat. It is much more difficult to inject Zyderm II through a 30-gauge needle. We sometimes use the 27-gauge needle for the 65% Zyderm II.

Successful correction with Zyderm collagen depends largely on the selection of suitable scars and wrinkles. In the same patient, some scars may respond favorably whereas others will not. The most responsive scars are small to large, soft scars with gently sloping sides. These can be identified by placing the thumb and index finger on each side of the scar and spreading the skin in opposite directions. If the surface of the scar comes into a flat plane with the skin surface, the scar will probably respond well. Hard, firm scars with almost perpendicular edges can be improved partially by repeated injections of Zyderm collagen. In such scars, initial injections often serve to soften the scar and allow for subsequent distention. Some scars, however, can be corrected to only 50% of their initial depth; these scars are probably best treated by surgical means such as dermabrasion. Scars least likely to respond are ice-pick scars for which punch replacement is preferred.

ACNE SCARS

For acne scars we use three injection techniques. In scars that can be gently but firmly held between the index finger and the thumb, we insert the needle tip 3.0–5.0 mm from the edge of the scar at a 20–45-degree angle. The needle is inserted into the skin and advanced slowly until an increase in resistance is felt, an indication that the bevel of the needle has entered the scar (Fig 9–5,A). The needle should now be in the upper or middermis. Zyderm collagen is slowly injected with firm pressure in an attempt to elevate the scar surface above the level of the surrounding skin. The scar should blanch white and appear as a small, white mound sometimes with an orange-peel effect after injection.

The amount of material injected varies with the size and firmness of the scar. During implantation, the scar may become elevated to a certain level at which additional injected material spreads laterally in the skin, causing no increased elevation of the scar. This indicates an end point for injection.

If the scar cannot be secured easily between the thumb and index finger, we then fixate the scar by pressing with the thumb and index finger on the adjacent skin. Starting 3.0–5.0 mm adjacent to the scar, we advance the needle until we feel the tip within the scar tissue and inject as described above. This technique of advancing the needle to gauge tissue resistance and thus to insure the needle is in the scar is analogous to a venipuncture in reverse. During venipuncture, there is an increased resistance as the needle is advanced, and upon entering the vein, there is a decreased resistance. Very helpful in this injection technique is to bend the needle 45 degrees before starting the injection. This does not impede flow of the collagen and keeps the bevel high in the dermis during advancement of the needle.

In very small scars, angling the needle at 45 degrees may place the bevel partly inside and partly outside the scar; as a result, more collagen may be extruded around the scar than into it. In this case, we inject directly into the middle of the scar perpendicular to the skin. Since most acne scars are atrophic, the needle should be advanced very slowly so that the bevel is just covered by the epidermis. If the needle is advanced rapidly, it may puncture the skin and deposit the implant material subcutaneously, where it has less beneficial effect.

We are not convinced that the direction of the needle bevel during injection—whether up, down, or sideways—has any bearing on treatment outcome. Nevertheless, we generally inject with the bevel up, using the 45-degree bend of the needle to stay high in the skin and to prevent puncture into the subcutaneous tissue. With the bevel up, we can see more easily whether it is in the skin.

Injection of acne scars can be facilitated by using a Lucite device or similar wider grip aid that slips over the prepackaged syringe (Fig 9–4). This device increases the leverage on the plunger by giving a wider finger grip than the standard, disposable, tuberculin-type syringe.

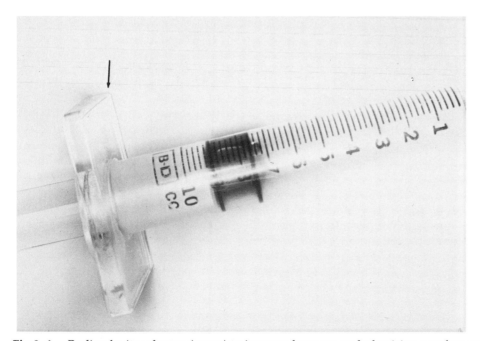

Fig 9–4.—Bodian lucite adaptor *(arrow)* to increase leverage and physician comfort on a disposable syringe.

Linear surgical scars are injected in the same fashion as acne scars. We start at one end of the scar and extrude Zyderm collagen once the bevel is fully in the skin. The lidocaine in the collagen dispersion produces some anesthesia. When the needle is advanced to the maximum length desired and then withdrawn. We always try to insert the needle into the previously injected, anesthetized area to diminish patient discomfort.

Atrophic scars that result from injections of intralesional corticosteroids require a different approach. Atrophic skin has lost most of its tensile strength. Therefore, overcorrection in these scars may tear superficial skin. We do not overcorrect atrophic corticosteroid-induced scars. Instead, we gradually implant small amounts of collagen over several treatment sessions to build the thickness and strength of the scar.

INJECTION OF WRINKLES, CREASES, AND FOLDS

In fine, early wrinkles such as those lateral to the nasolabial fold or in the midcheek area, we pinch the skin between the index finger and thumb and inject linearly high in the dermis. We inject Zyderm collagen in front of the advancing needle point to limit the needle prick discomfort, and, if necessary, add additional Zyderm collagen as we withdraw the needle. For deeper wrinkles, particularly in thick skin, we use the double-layer injection technique (Fig 9–5,B). Here, Zyderm collagen is deposited linearly in the deep dermis or dermal-fat junction. A second line of Zyderm collagen then is deposited high into the dermis to cause significant overcorrection. Gentle massage is needed to eliminate the blanching. We think that gentle massage may result in a more even dispersion of Zyderm collagen throughout skin, affording a better clinical outcome. We have no scientific evidence, however, and no formal bilateral comparison study has yet been done to support this premise. The gentle massage leaves the patient's skin looking less bumpy, and patients who have received it after injection generally request massage in subsequent treatment sessions.

Another technique for injecting early superficial creases and wrinkles is to puncture the skin multiple times along the axis of the wrinkle (Fig 9–6,A and B). The physician's free hand is placed on the patient's skin around the wrinkle and stretches the skin and stabilizes it. The syringe is then rested on the physician's thumb and rocked into position so that the bevel of the needle just barely penetrates the high dermis in the area of the crease. The bevel can be up or down depending on how deep the material is going to be planted. Multiple penetrations are made, with tiny amounts of collagen injected at each site. Sometimes, when the skin is so porous that the material easily escapes or when a crease does not elevate equally, multiple punctures can be made with the needle held perpendicular to the axis of the crease. Both this multiple puncture technique and the threading technique are valuable, and each physician will learn by experience when to use a given technique. Sometimes all techniques are required to elevate the crease to the desired level.

A Depressed scars

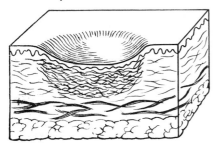
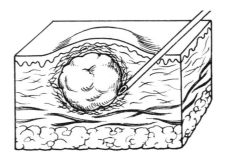

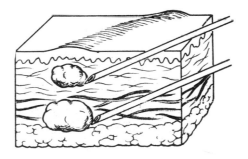

B Wrinkles and creases

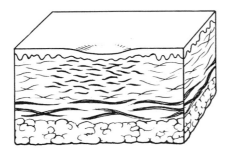
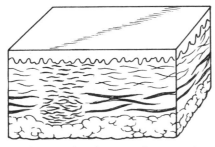

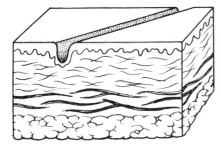

Fig 9–5.—A, injection technique for depressed scars, tip of needle enters center of scar. **B,** double-layer injection technique, one injection into the deep dermis and a second, superficial to the first, into the papillary dermis.

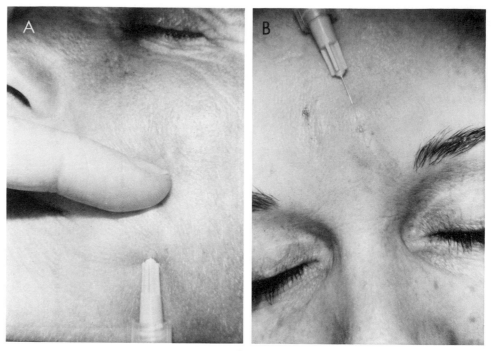

Fig 9–6.—Injection of Zyderm collagen implant.

INJECTION OF THE UPPER LIP

We use two techniques to inject the upper lip. The first is for the patient whose wrinkles are primarily at the vermilion border without extending into the upper part of the upper lip. The 30-gauge needle is inserted into the vermilion line at the lateral edge of the lip, and the Zyderm collagen is slowly extruded. When the needle tip is in the proper space, the Zyderm collagen advances toward the center of the lip in worm-like fashion, but is confined to the vermilion border and thus to the area of wrinkles. The needle is withdrawn and then inserted toward the middle of the lip into the area already containing Zyderm collagen. Insertion into an anesthetized area minimizes the discomfort of a new needle prick on the upper lip. The same process is continued farther along the vermilion if needed. Often, three injections suffice for early wrinkles at the vermilion border, and the patient feels only one needle prick.

If the patient has wrinkles at the vermilion that extend into the upper portion of the upper lip, we inject the vermilion as described and inject each wrinkle on the lip by entering through the Zyderm-anesthetized area. A linear mass of Zyderm collagen is placed high into the superficial dermis into each wrinkle.

For the older patient who has a shriveled-looking upper lip. Here, the whole upper lip needs to be built up. Since large volumes and greater numbers of needle pricks are involved, we occasionally do bilateral infraorbital nerve blocks to anesthetize the entire upper lip. Zyderm collagen can then be injected intradermally and subdermally without discomfort.

INJECTION OF GLABELLAR LINES

When the patient is supine, glabellar lines may be difficult to see, and over-hang problems may not be appreciated. Thus, glabellar folds are usually best injected with the patient semi-upright on an examination table. We stand at the head of the table and reach over the top of the patient's head to inject the lines. This procedure can be done in reverse; however, the curve of the nose and cheeks often prevents as accurate an injection. When injecting from below, the 45-degree bend of the needle is very helpful. Since the arteries of the central face can connect with the intracranial vessels. Special care must be taken to inject only into the dermis. No injection should be below the dermis and if the needle should pass completely through the skin, stop injecting at once.

NASOLABIAL FOLDS

Three injection techniques are used:

For very early wrinkles with little depth, a series of individual high intradermal injections along the line works well. The elevated areas should be massaged so that the collagen material is evenly distributed.

For the patient with deeper wrinkles, early creasing, and without overhang of the cheeks, the double-layer technique for injecting wrinkles is used providing the skin is thick enough. Excellent results can be obtained by injecting two levels linearly throughout the nasolabial-meilolabial line.

In the patient whose folds are due to overhang of the cheeks, Zyderm collagen is injected into the upper lip adjacent to the nasolabial fold. Then, with finger pressure and slight massage, the material is worked into the nasolabial-meilolabial fold area. We try to decrease the contrast of the high cheek and low lip by building up the lateral lip. Injecting the nasolabial folds in a patient with overhanging skin theoretically puts half of the material into the overhanging portion of the cheek, limiting the cosmetic benefit. If most of the material were injected into the overhanging portion of the cheek, the patient's appearance might actually be worsened by accentuating the high-low contrast of these adjacent structures. It is important to evaluate how much is actual creasing due to sun damage and muscular action and how much is due to cheek overhang secondary to sagging of the cheek.

CROW'S-FEET

Crow's-feet wrinkles lateral to the lateral border of the bony orbit can be injected with satisfactory results. Tiny amounts of Zyderm collagen are injected linearly into each wrinkle. Massage is very important here to disperse the injected material evenly through the skin. We stop at the bony orbit and do not inject into eyelid tissue. The thinness of eyelid tissue and the relatively large volume of Zyderm collagen going into this tissue can produce a lumpy look. Theoretically, it should be possible to correct eyelid wrinkles by injecting minute amounts of Zyderm collagen and then massaging. However, at this time we have not developed the proficiency to recommend a specific technique and we personally avoid injecting into eyelid tissue.

FOREHEAD WRINKLES

Depending on the depth and thickness of skin, forehead wrinkles can be injected intradermally, linearly, or by the double-layer injection technique previously described. One can obtain excellent results when the face is in repose. However, the frontalis muscle reinstitutes some of these wrinkles during animated speech. Thus, the physician and patient must decide if the improvement during repose and partial improvement during speech is of sufficient benefit.

OTHER WRINKLES

Fine lines on the cheek are particularly responsive to therapy when the implant material is placed high in the dermis. However, deep creases and severe sagging in sun-damaged skin are often best corrected with a face peel or dermabrasion and occasionally with a face-lift. For many fine wrinkles in the motivated patient, however, Zyderm implant therapy is worthwhile.

A variety of other lines can be injected with either the intradermal or the double-layer technique. These include chin lines, linear scars above the eyebrows, linear nose wrinkles and neck wrinkles.

Minor facial contouring can be done to make the malar eminences or the chin slightly more prominent. Here the double-layer injection technique is used, and the Zyderm collagen is molded with the fingers to confine it to the desired area of augmentation. Molding or massaging the material into the correct contours is vital for the patient to be satisfied with the result. The molding effects seem to be lost sooner in these areas than in scars and wrinkles, however.

The patient is advised that there may be some bruising in the area and there may be some minor persistent palpable alteration for the first four or five days. Retreatment can be as early as two weeks but can be at any time after that.

We have found that far less material is required (thus, at lower cost to the patient) if we are careful to inject in the upper dermal region and create a blanched, elevated appearance immediately after the injection. It is difficult to estimate how many treatments and how much material will be needed until one has had considerable experience with the use of Zyderm. As an extremely gross estimate for those patients with moderate soft acne scarring, 1.0 ml will treat all of the lesions at a given sitting, and usually three to four sittings are necessary. For treating creases and wrinkles, the nasolabial crease often requires 1.0 ml on each side of the face per sitting whereas, for the quite fine secondary creases that occur lateral to the nasolabial crease and extend onto the chin, as well as those fine creases around the mouth, 1.0 ml often will be sufficient at a given sitting.

SELECTION OF PATIENTS

Patients with ice-pick postacne scars or extremely tiny, deeply depressed scars often are not selected for Zyderm implants if any other modality is available. If it is believed that they will not respond to dermabrasion or punch transplant, they can be treated with Zyderm, but only a small percentage will benefit. Patients who have soft, pliable scars with gently sloping edges are the best candidates.[6] Many patients have a variety of postacne scars and must be

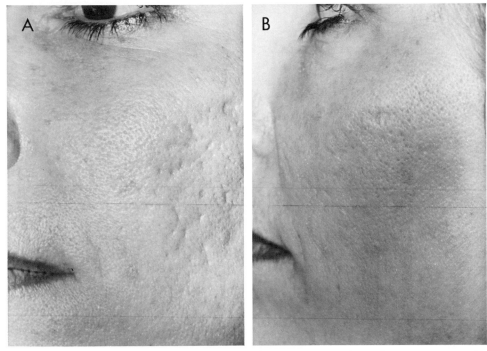

Fig 9–7.—A, thirty-six-year-old woman with postacne scarring prior to treatment. **B,** after 3 treatments with Zyderm collogen. Approximately 1.5 ml used on each cheek.

reminded that certain types of scars will respond to certain types of treatments and that each scar will have to be individualized. We try first to use the modality that will reduce most of the scars and then touch up with a second modality. For example, if patients have severe ice-pick scarring, we may do punch transplants and dermabrasion, and then later use Zyderm for a few of the depressions. However, if the depressed scars are the most numerous or cosmetically unacceptable scars, we use Zyderm first, offering full-face or spot dermabrasion later as needed.

Patients who have a great many soft, undulating scars over a large portion of the cheeks (Fig 9–7), temples, and forehead (Fig 9–8) have not responded as well as we had hoped. Although the scars are depressed and soft and seem to elevate easily with the injection of the Zyderm, we seem to "get lost" between visits, and the patient never ends up with smooth skin. Although there is visible improvement and all agree that the scars look better, there will still be significant, obvious acne scarring. Our best results are for patients who have fewer scars with a greater amount of normal tissue between the scars.

We also have been able to improve the texture of fibrotic scars, although we have not been able to improve as much of the superficial irregularity. This was a benefit of the implant that was not predicted but clearly one that we and the patients could observe. It is difficult to inject into fibrotic scars, but with use of the 30-gauge needle and the handle extender, a fair amount of collagen can be worked, over several visits, into the thickened fibrotic scars. They begin to soften, and the texture of the face has a better feel. We do not recommend the procedure to many patients, since the material is relatively expensive and the

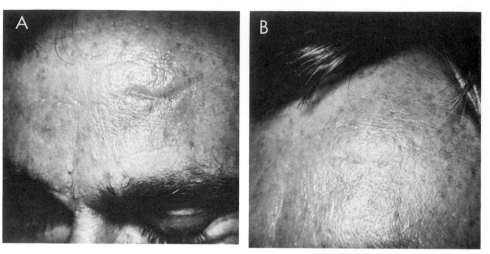

Fig 9–8.—A, forty-two-year-old man with posttraumatic and postacne scarring, forehead, prior to treatment. **B,** four months after the last treatment of Zyderm collagen injections, 2 ml total injected.

contour of the face is not actually changed by this technique. However, when injecting other types of scars, it often is helpful to "soften" some of the fibrotic scars.

Certain age lines or sun-damaged skin lines respond very well, some better than others. We have found that the nasolabial and meilolabial lines, if they are dermal creases and not thick, overhanging cheek skin, respond very well (Fig 9–9). The response is better on the more inferior portion of these creases around the sides of the mouth and at the level of the mustache. The secondary meilolabial lines, which form lateral to the main meilolabial line, respond extremely well. Treatment of these lines is particularly helpful for the patient in the late 30s, early 40s, and 50s who has not developed many other signs of aging but has these telltale marks on the central cheeks. Sometimes only one injection is necessary to correct completely these secondary nasolabial lines for

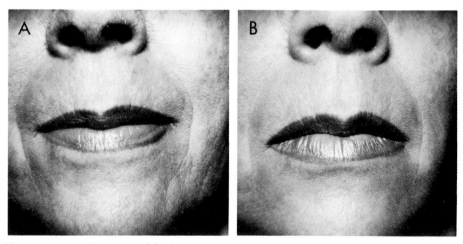

Fig 9–9.—A, deep nasolabial creases in a forty-five-year-old woman. **B,** three months after third treatment with Zyderm collagen implant, total of 6 ml used.

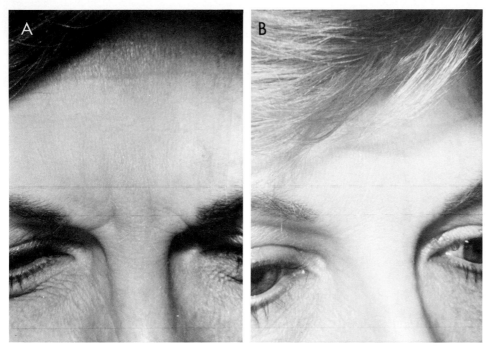

Fig 9–10.—A, thirty-eight-year-old woman with vertical glabellar creases prior to treatment. **B,** two months after second injection of Zyderm collagen, total of 2 ml used. (Patient bleached hair after successful improvement with Zyderm collagen.)

many, many months. The vertical glabellar creases seem to respond best of all of the facial lines (Fig 9–10). Sometimes only one treatment is necessary to correct completely some of these creases, although two or three treatments are usual. The vertical radial lines of the upper lip also respond well, but if there are multiple creases, the patient is probably a better candidate for a dermabrasion or face peeling. For women who are just beginning to get some of the wrinkles of the vermilion border of the upper lip, small amounts of Zyderm can be injected by passing the needle along the dermal-epidermal junction the full length of the vermilion border. As the needles traverse the skin, small amounts of collagen can be confined to the area of the vermilion border that pushes out or puffs out these wrinkles. It does not distort the lip if done carefully; it enhances the vermilion or pink portion of the lip show and decreases the visibility of these wrinkles. It will stop some of the running of the lipstick, which is a very difficult problem for these patients.

The radial creases of the lower lip respond somewhat but not as much as the upper lip.

The horizontal forehead lines also are good lines for treatment, but, as mentioned above, care must be taken not to overinject these. The crow's feet or the small wrinkle lines at the corners of the eyes respond best lateral to the orbital rim and, with difficulty, medial to the orbital rim. This very thin tissue shows the collagen injection for a long time. We try to limit our injections of the crow's feet to only those lateral to the orbital rim and only after we have carefully discussed the situation with the patient. Neck creases also do very well, with high patient satisfaction, although the injected sites are detectable.

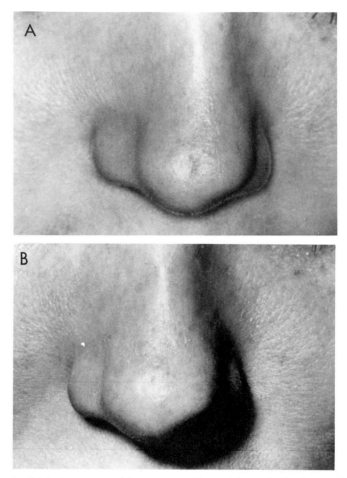

Fig 9–11.—A, thirty-two-year-old woman with postrhinoplasty depression of the nasal tip. **B,** three months after the fifth injection of Zyderm collagen, total of 2.5 ml used.

Another use that has proved to be helpful is in the small overhang of the upper lip over the lower that occurs in some patients. This seems to be a hereditary fold that can be pushed out with several injections of collagen at the lateral commissures. The overhang seems to correct enough that the chronic perlèche that tends to develop there is alleviated. We also have found collagen to be helpful in some fibrotic and depressed scars. They did not improve clinically, but the direction of the whiskers improved enough that the patient was greatly relieved in his shaving habits. Formerly, these irregularly directed whiskers would grow into the skin, creating a small and persistent sore, whereas after collagen injections it no longer was true.

There are many other conditions for which Zyderm collagen injection has been used: postrhinoplasty depressions, traumatic defects, depressed surgical scars (Fig 9–11), depressed split-thickness skin grafts, facial hemiatrophy, etc. However, the percentage of improvement of these types of lesions that respond to Zyderm is more variable than that of soft, depressed acne scarring and small, fine facial wrinkling.

Zyderm II 65% has just become available and is very popular. We have used it in the early clinical trials. We predict that some physicians will use it almost exclusively; others seldom; and most of us will use both Zyderm I 35% and Zyderm II 65%. With experience clear preferences may emerge. The smaller syringe makes injection easier than with Zyderm I.

We like to think that Zyderm collagen is an excellent way to correct dermal defects. In our mind's eye, we envision the tip of our 30-gauge needle in the dermis, either deep or superficial, for in that area the retention of the correction seems to last the longest. In those few cases in which we have had the opportunity to obtain biopsy specimens in human beings, the collagen dispersed in and among the native collagen fibers seems to have adapted perfectly and, indeed, been accepted by the host. When we have injected into the subcutaneous tissues, the correction was short-lived and often completely lost. When we think of using collagen to mold or shape thick, fibrotic, or "heavy" depressed lesions, we generally have been less successful.

The long-term retention of the correction is difficult to evaluate at this point. When we originally used the material, we used it on many lesions, and some of those treatments have proved to be ineffective. This, of course, affects our long-term success negatively. Currently, we are using it on both static lesions, such as scars, and dynamic lesions, such as wrinkles and creases. Originally, we hoped that the correction of these defects would be permanent. But as we follow patients for several years, the obvious change in the face is more apparent or at least is brought to our attention, and we are not sure now that we really desire a permanent implant. The Collagen Corporation has released evidence that indicates that for static scars, such as a depressed acne scar, the clinical improvement will tend to regress to about 80% of its best level and remain that way for two to three years. This is the limit of our long-term follow-up at the present date. Retention of correction has been found in a high percentage of those lesions that originally were deemed appropriate. We believe that our treatment of creases and wrinkles, in the way that we now see as proper, will last for 6–9 months. However, touch-up treatments require less material.

The concept of an impermanent implant is new for us. We see evidence of lasting correction of a defect and cannot be sure whether it is the implant or the implant replaced by native collagen responsible for the lasting correction. Also by definition a "replaceable" implant will be subject to the natural variations in patients and variation of stability within certain anatomic areas.

ADVERSE REACTIONS

In data released in 1982 by the Collagen Corporation on adverse reactions, there were 284 positive test site responses of 9,427 patients, or a 3% incidence. The greatest percent of these test site responses involved only the test site where there was a combination of erythema, induration, swelling, pruritus, and tenderness. As mentioned above, more than 70% of these sites were positive within the first 72 hours. From this group of patients, 34 responses were both localized and systemic, the systemic reaction including arthralgia, generalized rash, generalized pruritis, myalgia, and 3 cases of a slight difficulty in breathing.

The untoward reactions from treatment sites have divided into two areas: associated treatment responses and adverse treatment responses. To our minds, the associated treatment responses are not more than could be expected from any intralesional injections. They include rupture of small vessels, inadvertent arterial spasm, and intermittent localized swelling and erythema. There have been some cases of ecchymoses followed by sloughing at the injection site. (This was mentioned above.)

The most serious problems with Zyderm collagen injection have been the adverse treatment responses—33 cases of 5,109 patients with a sensitization manifested by localized swelling, induration, pruritus, or erythema at the treatment site following a response-free test dose. These are the patients who were skin-test–negative and later became allergic to the material. These erythematous and indurated reactions at treatment sites have been a nuisance to manage, since they are usually on the face and persist between 4 and 11 months. Thus far, there have been a few systemic reactions of the erythema multiforme type in patients who had a negative test site and then later became allergic. The management for these late allergic responses has been symptomatic only. Intralesional and systemic corticosteroids help some of the symptoms and help reduce the amount of visible erythema and induration. However, the reaction seems to last for 5–11 months and eventually resolves. Interestingly, 90% of late allergic reactions occur within the first month of treatment.

Data compiled on large populations of patients shows a similar number of reactions: about 3% allergic to the skin test and about .3%–.4% develop an aquired allergy. There has been one reported case of unilateral blindness following a Zyderm collagen injection into verticle wrinkles of the forehead. This unfortunate event underscores the need to keep the injections high in the dermis.

CONCLUSION

We have been pleased with the opportunity to use Zyderm collagen in its initial studies, and we continue to use it on a regular basis in our practice. It has not only enhanced our ability to treat postacne scarring, but also has led us to offer therapy to more and more patients, since the combined use of Zyderm collagen, dermabrasion, and punch transplants all help us improve the appearance of enough patients to make it worth their effort. We are especially gratified to have a treatment for patients who develop creases and wrinkles at an early age. Men and women who look like they are scowling or frowning or who have the premature, isolated wrinkles and creases can be helped by this relatively simple and inexpensive manner. The alternatives to date have been surgical intervention that usually was fairly complicated, such as a coronal approach for a forehead lift or a complete rhytidectomy, or dermabrasion and chemical peeling, which also are fairly extensive procedures.

On the other hand, we cannot caution too much that this is a new product, and it will be many years before we know the full ramifications of our work. We never encourage a patient to have Zyderm injections if he or she has not been fully advised of the potential and unknown risks. If the patient shows any hesitation, we will not give an injection, since it will lead to worry on the patient's part for many years. We discuss the adverse reactions of which we are aware. We also tell them that we always must act in a conservative way that is in the patient's best interest. Most of the time, collagen injections are used for a benign or cosmetic problem, and this benefit must be carefully measured against any potential risk.

REFERENCES

1. Knapp T.R., Luck E., Daniels J.R.: Behavior of solubilized collagen as a bioimplant. *J. Surg. Res.* 23:96-105, 1977.
2. Knapp T.R., Kaplan E.N., Daniels J.R.: Injectable collagen for soft tissue augmentation. *Plast. Reconstr. Surg.* 60:39-45, 1977.
3. Report of the Initial California Cooperative Study Group (Daniels J.R., Falces E., Fisher W., et al.), October 1979. On file at Collagen Corp., Palo Alto, Calif.
4. Barr R.J., King D.F., McDonald R.M., et al.: Necrobiotic granulomas associated with bovine collagen test site injections. *J. Am. Acad. Dermatol.* 6:867–869, 1982.
5. Collagen Corporation. Summary of Clinical Investigation. February 1982, Palo Alto, Calif.
6. Stegman S.J., Tromovitch T.A.: Implantation of collagen for depressed scars. *J. Dermatol. Surg. Oncol.* 6:450–453, 1980.

10 / Tattoo Removal

EXCISION AND PRIMARY CLOSURE is the single best method of removing tattoos because it consistently removes all of the tattoo and produces one of the best cosmetic results. The tattoo is excised through a full-thickness excision of skin, including a small amount of subcutaneous fat. Because most tattoos are on the extremities or trunk, the patient should be informed that a spread scar is being substituted for a tattoo; a spread scar may be the best result the patient can expect. The patient also should be warned that sometimes unsightly or keloidal scars develop. Fine-line results after excising significant amounts of skin on the trunk or extremities does not happen consistently.

Where a single elliptical excision would not encompass the entire tattoo, would result in an excessively long scar, or would produce excess tension on the wound edges, serial excisions can be undertaken (Fig 10–1). First, the center of the tattoo is excised, taking out that width of tissue consistent with good surgical judgment. The skin is allowed to loosen—usually for 12–24 weeks or even longer. The scar and the remainder of the tattoo then are excised at a second sitting. Sometimes a third excision is necessary for complete removal or for a better cosmetic result.

A useful approach for the final serial excision is to take up the tension across the wound with buried, interrupted, sutures; then place a running subcuticular Prolene suture. Since Prolene has so little reactivity, the suture can be left in for three or four weeks to give the wound sufficient time to gain strength. This will greatly reduce the chance of dehiscence. Rarely is there a reaction to Prolene left in for several weeks, and it can be removed easily because of its slick monofilament construction.

Sometimes a tattoo has an unusual configuration so that it cannot be encompassed easily within an ellipse. In such cases, various configurations are possible. These include curvilinear or S-shaped excisions, stellate excisions, multiple ellipses at different angles to one another, and triangular excisions. In other cases a small flap, such as a rotation flap or transposition flap, will produce the best possible scar. It might be necessary to excise an entire tattoo and plan to cover this large defect with a split-thickness skin graft. The graft does not necessarily produce a cosmetically acceptable result and it does produce a second donor defect. However, if the site of the donor defect is chosen carefully, e.g., the lateral buttocks in the bathing suit area, some patients are happy to trade their tattoo for a graft and a hidden donor site.

The advantage of the excision methods is that the tattoo is entirely removed and the result is the type of scar that might have been caused by trauma or an excision of a cutaneous lesion. The result can be passed off as the scar from an accident or from the "wise" excision of a previously existing lesion. This is in sharp contrast to some of the other modalities that we describe below.

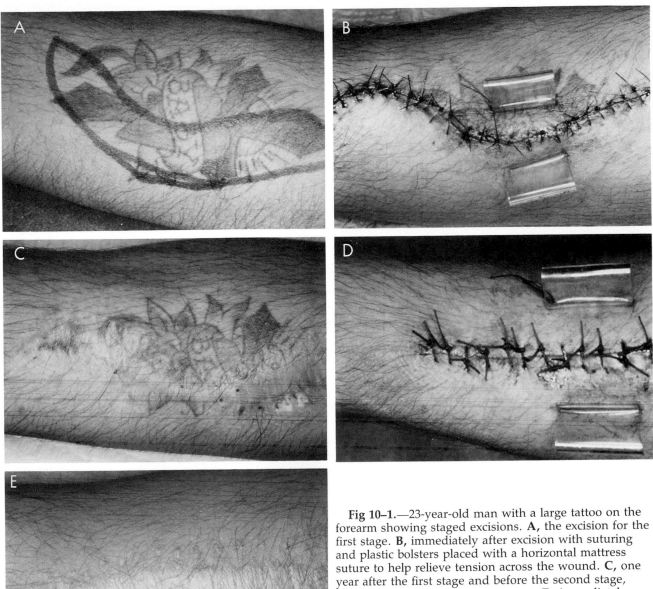

Fig 10–1.—23-year-old man with a large tattoo on the forearm showing staged excisions. **A,** the excision for the first stage. **B,** immediately after excision with suturing and plastic bolsters placed with a horizontal mattress suture to help relieve tension across the wound. **C,** one year after the first stage and before the second stage, which removes the remaining tattoo. **D,** immediately after the second stage of removal, sutured again with interrupted sutures and plastic bolsters with a horizontal mattress suture. **E,** one year after the second stage excision and complete healing.

SCARIFICATION

Folklore tells us that some American Indian tribes made multiple small linear superficial incisions in their skin over a tattoo. Goat's milk was applied and the area bandaged with a cloth. The tattoo pigment would be drawn into the eschar and caught up with this crust. Goat's milk was said to be the most effective way of attracting the pigment. But since that time, it has been shown that almost any eschar formation will collect a great deal of pigment. Whether this is secondary to inflammation or is a normal transepidermal elimination process of healing never has been completely worked out. Prisoners also have treated themselves with razor blades and produced similar scarification. In 1888 Variot described a similar method by using linear incisions, scratches, or punctures in the skin over the tattoo.[1] The French method involved the application of tannic acid and silver nitrate to create a very thick eschar.[2] This eschar also caused a great deal of sloughing of the pigment.

More recently, tannic acid and silver nitrate application has been added to a superficial dermabrasion with standard diamond chip fraises. The method, popularized by Penhoff, involves applying tannic acid solution to the tattoo and then lightly dermabrading the area. The dermabrasion plus the tannic acid makes a slurry of foam and cutaneous debris. This is carefully wiped off, and the procedure is repeated. Following the two slurries, silver nitrate sticks are rubbed over the wound and a thick, tenacious, flexible crust forms. When this crust finally separates, there is a significant loss of the pigment from the tattoo. This method is also being used by some military physicians today, with good results reported. The tannic acid formula is: 2 parts tannic acid, 1 part glycerin, and 1 part distilled water.

SALABRASION

This is another method that arose in antiquity.[3] Whether it truly started with a Greek physician named Aëtius half a century after the death of Christ or whether it was a common practice of South Pacific island natives is academic. One of the first medical papers on this method was written in the German literature in 1935.[4] Recent interest in salabrasion started in the early 1970s. Several papers recorded the methods that produced good results and even the histologic correlation with clinical results.[5–7]

To perform salabrasion, a simple abrading apparatus is necessary. It can be a wooden doorknob or any other solid object. Then a 4x4-in. gauze is fashioned around this handle and the gauze is wet in ordinary tap water and dipped into table salt. The tattoo can be anesthetized with Xylocaine, but the hypertonic saline slurry that soon results also is anesthetic. The tattoo is held taut by four-point traction and the area abraded vigorously until it turns bright red. It is important to carry on the salabrasion through glistening and light pinkness to the heavy, blood-red appearance. It also is important to have this depth of abrasion throughout the entire area of the tattoo. During the process, a hypertonic saline solution is created at the surface of the skin. The present-day theory on the effectiveness of the method is that the solution creates a chemotactic factor for phagocytes. Sometimes the salt is left on and a dressing is applied; at other times, the salt is washed away and a dressing is applied.

Variations of salabrasion use rock salt instead of table salt, and there are a multitude of different "favorite" dressings applied.

Most of the time, a simple gentian violet or antibiotic-impregnated dressing is applied and a crust or eschar is allowed to form. This then is treated in fashion standard for any superficial abrasion type of injury.

The results in some cases are truly excellent,[8] and the simplicity and low morbidity make the procedure attractive to many physicians. As could be expected, however, the results often are similar to that of superficial dermabrasion and have led to atrophic or hypertrophic scars, irregular loss of pigmentation, and some complete failures. Physicians who perform both superficial dermabrasion and salabrasion have difficulty in relating what technique variables may produce more salutary results. If salabrasion is used for smaller lesions with the patient understanding that excision may be required later, it is a good simple method to try initially.

SUPERFICIAL DERMABRASION

The area can be anesthetized in standard fashion by local infiltration or with field block Xylocaine or it can be frozen with Freon 112, ethyl chloride, or any of the other refrigerants. Freezing of the skin is not necessary. Some surgeons prefer to hold the skin taut with four-point traction and dermabrade under full visualization, without the encumbrance of the frosting.

In this technique, a diamond fraise is used to abrade only the epidermis down to the level of the papillary dermis.[9] No attempt is made to remove all the pigment as is done with other methods that will be discussed below. This depth can be recognized clinically because of the regular pinpoint bleeding that will show up after the frost has completely dissipated. Another way to recognize this level is by the stippled appearance of the skin.

Hemostasis is obtained with pressure or with applications of styptics such as 30% aluminum chloride in alcohol. The wound is covered with gentian violet and an appropriately sized dressing, made with either Telfa or Adaptic. An eschar forms, and sometimes the pigment will migrate into the eschar or into the nonstick dressing. Good examples are on record in which the exact pattern of the tattoo was found on the dressing or on the reverse side of the eschar. Whether the gentian violet plays an important part in this procedure never has been documented, since the same types of results have been obtained with other types of dressings. The theory that the gentian violet stimulated movement of the pigment-containing macrophages of skin also never has been proved.

The results of superficial dermabrasion, as with other techniques, are variable. Some results are excellent, showing little change in the skin after this type of dermabrasion. Others report that one, two, or three additional dermabrasions are necessary before adequate amounts of pigment are extruded from the skin. Unfortunately, even with a superficial abrasion, there have been reported cases of hypopigmentation and hyperpigmentation, hypertrophic scarring, and irregular success with tattoo elimination. Thus far, we are not aware of good criteria in selecting patients for this technique. We agree to do this procedure if the patient wants it and will agree to later excision if the results are not satisfactory.

WIRE BRUSH DERMABRASION

Wire brush dermabrasion was used more commonly in the 1950s and 1960s and was especially successful for tattoos on the face. It also was acceptable for traumatic tattoos where the material was embedded at various layers in the skin. The standard technique with a wire brush involves local anesthesia of the skin, followed by an extremely hard freeze with any one of the standard refrigerants.[10, 11] The brush then is used to remove the tattoo pigment from the dermis. Refreezing often is necessary so that gouging or running of the wire brush on unfrozen skin is less likely. A dermabrasion is carried to the level of the dermis where only tiny dots of tattoo pigment remain. The dots then are removed manually, using magnification, with fine forceps and scissors or with a curet. After all of the pigment has been removed, a dressing is placed with an antibiotic ointment and the wound is followed carefully. With newer dressings, such as Biobrane and Op-Site, it might be possible to encourage quicker healing with less hypertrophic scarring. However, these materials have not been used often enough after dermabrasion for us to make any specific recommendations.

The problem with this technique is that on the face it often is successful whereas on the extremities there is a high incidence of hypertrophic scarring. With the use of this method, it is important to make an abrasion wound that is in a different geometric pattern and, thus to disguise the fact that a tattoo had existed. To have a tattoo in the shape of a bird or snake treated and then produce a hypertrophic scar in exactly the same shape does not give the needed cosmetic improvement. By creating an oval, circular, or other geometric form, the patient can give other excuses for the etiology of the scar.

Tattoos that are done professionally usually are placed with the pigment residing just under the epidermis for several months. As the tattoo ages, the phagocytes engulf the pigment and migrate more deeply into the dermis. Consequently, for old tattoos, particularly on the face, the wire brush dermabrasion often is recommended. For more recent tattoos, a superficial diamond fraise type of dermabrasion has a good chance for success, with less chance for development of a hypertrophic scar.

SPLIT-THICKNESS TANGENTIAL EXCISION

One of the machines, such as the Brown dermatome or the Davol, can be used to take a split-thickness section of skin from the tattoo area and then dress the wound as one would after a standard split-thickness removal or with gentian violet, with the hope that this may increase the amount of pigment-containing phagocytes migrating into the dressing.[12] These instruments allow the physician to remove a preselected thickness of skin, which may or may not lead to less scarring during healing. Again, the evidence is mixed because there are some cases reported with excellent results and minimal or no scarring whereas at other times, particularly on the extremities, the area will also develop irregular hypertrophic and irregularly pigmented scars. This is a good technique for large tattoos, where it is hard to excise and close primarily or excise in staged excisions.

LASERS[14–16]

Originally it was believed that the ruby lasers would be a good treatment of tattoos because of their affinity for the red pigment so often used in many tattoos. Even at best, this method is limited to that particular color.

More recently, the carbon dioxide laser, which can be set at either a cutting or vaporizing mode, is able to create a wound at a specific depth. For tattoos it usually is set at 100 μ deep. On the vaporizing mode, pulses of light are applied to the skin and can be carefully traced over the tattoo itself. Although this technique minimizes the overall wounding, the result is that the scar often is exactly the same shape as the original tattoo; exchanging a tattoo for a scar shaped like a bird or a snake, etc. More recent work involves the laser's being applied in a different geometric form over the tattoo, which results in an oval or circular scar. The results of laser treatment are very similar to those from a deep dermabrasion performed with either a diamond fraise or a wire brush.[17] Although there have been some excellent results after the carbon dioxide laser, there also have been hypertrophic scars, irregularly pigmented lesions, and wounds that were not completely free from pigment. With results and risks similar to those of dermabrasion, laser therapy still is too expensive and experimental to be recommended for a routine office setting. If one is available, it is a good alternative.

RETATTOOING

Using a flesh-colored pigment or white titanium dioxide, a professional tattoo artist can tattoo over an old tattoo. This highly placed pigment then will reflect light out of the skin without revealing the other pigments that are deeper. This effectively masks the appearance of the tattoo. However, flesh-colored pigment is only one color and never changes as does the patient's surrounding skin, which varies with exposure to the sun, vascular flushing, and skin temperature. As is so well known with the superficial fungus *Malassezia furfur*, spots on the skin that do not change color with sun or with vascular lability are quite obvious most of the time. Another technique with retattooing that does not change the tattoo and does not remove it or hide it is one that simply alters the shape, appearance, or lettering of a tattoo. Nude bodies can be clothed, names can be changed, and the stigmas of certain gangs can be covered with less offensive or more benign-appearing tattoos. For patients who do not mind the fact that they have a tattoo or do not like a specific tattoo, this often is the treatment of choice, since eradication by any of the above mentioned methods can cause unacceptable scarring.

CONCLUSION

The patient consultation about removal of tattoos is an extremely important part of this surgery. It often is helpful for the physician to try to understand why the patient wants the tattoo removed. These tattoos may remind the patient of an unhappy event or time or of hostility toward a person. Often the hostility is transferred to the physician. A resulting unsightly scar from treatment then is just the focus the patient needed (as well as the lawyers) to avoid facing the real event surrounding the placement of that tattoo.[18]

We believe that the single best method for removal is excision and primary closure. Many other methods have been documented in the popular literature as well as in the medical literature. We have tried, and still use, many of the other methods. We do so only with the patient's understanding that if the results are not satisfactory, excision should be considered.

If there were any way to predict when superficial or deep dermabrasion or salabrasion or tannic acid salabrasion would give good results rather than hypertrophic or irregularly pigmented scars, we are sure that these methods would be used more commonly by us. However, the one predictable scar is that from simple elliptical excision or excision using various forms of flaps. Once the patient understands what is going to happen, the results are at least satisfactory, if not completely successful, with excision and primary closure.

REFERENCES

1. Variot G.: Nouveau procede de destruction des tatouages. *C. R. Soc. Biol. (Paris)* 8:836-838, 1888.
2. Penhoff J.: The so-called French method of Variot. *J. Dermatol. Surg. Oncol.* 5:901-902, 1979.
3. Berchon E.: *Histoire Medicale du Tatouage.* Paris, J.B. Bailliere et Fils, 1869.
4. Klövekorn G.H.: Eine einfache methode der entfernung von tätowierungen. *Dermatol. Wochenschr.* 101:1271-1275, 1935.
5. Manchester G.H.: Tattoo removal. A new simple technique. *Calif. Med.* 118(3):10-12, 1973.
6. Crittenden F.M., Jr.: Salabrasion—removal of tattoos by superficial abrasion with table salt. *Cutis* 7:295-300, 1971.
7. Koerber W.A., Jr., Price N.M.: Salabrasion of tattoos. A correlation of the clinical and histological results. *Arch. Dermatol.* 114:884-888, 1978.
8. Price N.: Salabrasion. *J. Dermatol. Surg. Oncol.* 5:905, 1979.
9. Clabaugh W.: Removal of tattoos by superficial dermabrasion. *Arch. Dermatol.* 98:515-521, 1968.
10. Boo-Chai K.: The decorative tattoo: its removal by dermabrasion. *Plast. Reconstr. Surg.* 32:559-563, 1963.
11. Ceilley R.I., Goldstein N.: Dermabrasion. *J. Dermatol. Surg. Oncol.* 5:905, 1979.
12. Wheeler E.S., Miller T.A.: Tattoo removal by split thickness tangential excision. *West. J. Med.* 124:272-275, 1976.
13. Zacarian S.A.: Cryosurgery in dermatology. In: Goldschmidt H. (ed.): *Physical Modalities in Dermatologic Therapy.* New York, Springer-Verlag, 1978, pp. 270-281.
14. Apfelberg D.B., Maser M.R., Lash H.: Argon laser treatment of cutaneous vascular abnormalities: progress report. *Ann. Plast. Surg.* 1:14-18, 1978.
15. Goldman L., et al.: Laser treatment of tattoos: a preliminary survey of three years' clinical experience. *J.A.M.A.* 201:841-844, 1967.
16. Goldman L.: Effects of new laser systems on the skin. *Arch. Dermatol.* 108:385-390, 1973.
17. Arello C.R., et al.: Tattoo removal: comparative study of six methods in the pig. *Plast. Reconstr. Surg.* 70:699-703, 1982.
18. Zimmerman M.C.: Suits for malpractice based on alleged unsightly scars resulting from removal of tattoos. *J. Dermatol. Surg. Oncol.* 5:911-912, 1979.

11 / Treatment of Keloids

SUCCESSFUL TREATMENT OF KELOIDS is related to selection of proper treatment and long-term follow-up, with retreatment as necessary. The success can be predicted somewhat by differentiating a true keloid from a hypertrophic scar. Keloids tend to overgrow the boundaries of the original injury, most frequently develop on the upper back and chest, shoulders, jaw, and ear lobes, and are more common in young patients with darker skin; e.g., black or Hispanic people. Occasionally a keloid will form after injuries to the skin (acne, trauma, or surgery) and during the patient's rapid growth phase in the teenage years. Burn wounds often lead to keloids in patients who otherwise would not have them.

Hypertrophic scars can occur anywhere, on patients of all ages, and sometimes are secondary to wounds poorly or not approximated and wounds closed under tension or with poor surgical design. Keloids and hypertrophic scars commonly develop in areas where the muscle pull across the wound is strong, such as on the deltoid area or the upper arm in muscular young men. Many individuals have a hereditary predilection for hypertrophic scarring or keloids. Hypertrophic scars respond fairly well to treatment (or time) whereas keloids almost always have a questionably poor prognosis. The older the keloid is the less responsive it is to therapy.

The mainstay of keloid therapy is a combination of surgery and intralesional corticosteroids.[1-8] Whenever possible, the keloids should be excised and the defect closed with the least possible tension across the wound. Appropriate surgical techniques include simple elliptical excision with wide undermining and careful reapproximation of the wound edges, proximal flaps, Z-plasty scar revisions, or "shelling out" of the fibrous keloid with the use of the resulting redundant skin for the closure (Fig 11–1). Unfortunately, the risk of a second keloid forming is 50% or more and sometimes that second keloid is larger than the one originally excised.

Extremely wide keloids can be shaved off with a scalpel or razor blade and not closed primarily. Shave excisions must be treated immediately and for prolonged periods with intralesional corticosteroids. Linear keloids or spheroidal keloidal masses (such as found in the ear lobes) can be excised and the scar revised simultaneously to reduce tension across the defect, thereby discouraging new keloid formation.

For intralesional injections, we use triamcinolone acetonide (Kenalog) diluted with plain lidocaine or physiologic saline to concentrations between 5 and 40 mg/ml. The injection should be made every three to six weeks for as long as necessary to obtain flattening of the keloid. Some physicians like to use triamcinolone hexacetonide (Aristospan). However, the crystals of this medication remain in the skin for many months, which makes reinjection with this or

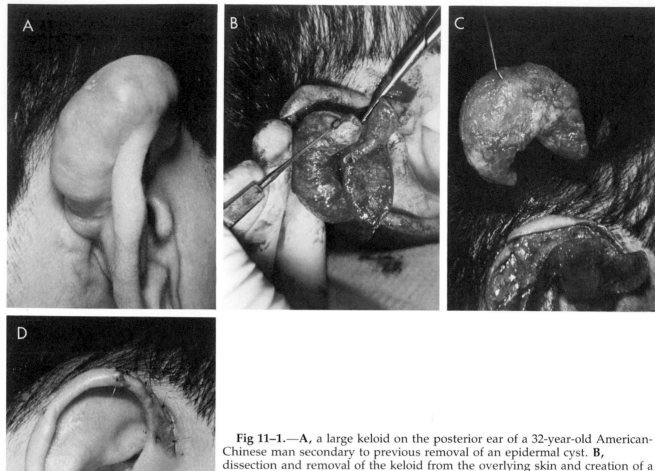

Fig 11–1.—A, a large keloid on the posterior ear of a 32-year-old American-Chinese man secondary to previous removal of an epidermal cyst. **B,** dissection and removal of the keloid from the overlying skin and creation of a flap from that excess skin. **C,** removal of the keloidal mass with the residual flap yet to be trimmed. **D,** final reshaping of the skin over the ear with suture closure.

other triamcinolones a calculated guess. The width and length of the keloidal scar will not be altered by the intralesional injections alone.

A 30-gauge needle on a disposable Luer-Lok® syringe is our favorite instrument for injecting keloids. A three-ring dental syringe also is comfortable for the physician's hand. There are disposable three-ring syringes or adapters available. The needle should be passed back and forth through the scar tissue to fill the entire keloid with medicine so that the surface blanches. A Dermojet sometimes is helpful for the initial softening of the outer portion of the keloid. These needleless injectors have different thrust strengths. It is important to know the way they are calibrated and the setting of your particular instrument. Usually for general dermatologic work, the penetration strength will allow only superficial penetration into firm keloids. However, if the keloid already is softened, a Dermojet may be adequate to penetrate the entire lesion. If there are no medical contraindications and the keloid is extremely firm, triamcinolone acetonide, 40 mg IM, will soften the keloid. This will permit easier intralesional injections two to three weeks later.

Liquid nitrogen cryotherapy 24 hours prior to intralesional injection helps the penetration of the steroid into the keloid. This probably is due to the interstitial edema of the freezing injury.[9]

Some patients experience severe pain during and after injection. For these patients, a field block using lidocaine 1% will prevent or alleviate the discomfort. As the keloids soften with repeated injection, pain lessens and the block may not be necessary.

Begin the injections with triamcinolone acetonide at lower concentrations (5 mg/ml) and increase the concentration slowly until softening or atrophy of the keloid occurs. If the lower concentrations do not produce a therapeutic response, gradually increase the concentration up to the full 40 mg/ml, remembering that triamcinolone crystals sometimes remain in the tissue longer than four weeks. Increasing the dose and injecting repeatedly without adequate time between injections leads to a build-up of triamcinolone crystals, possibly leading to overtreatment and prolonged atrophy around the lesion. Some patients are extremely sensitive and atrophy develops quickly even at lower concentrations. Repeated injections beneath the skin or even in nearby normal skin also will cause atrophy and worsen the appearance of the keloid. Unintentional injection or diffusion of the steroid into the surrounding skin and subcutaneous fat make long-acting triamcinolone hexacetonide (Aristospan) less acceptable.

When injecting the area where a keloid was excised, infiltrate the triamcinolone acetonide around the suture line. The first injection can be given immediately after the wound is closed or one week postoperatively. Some physicians prefer to inject a few days prior to excision. Continue these injections throughout the healing phase, at three-week intervals, until the wound shows no sign of keloid development. The wound should be watched carefully for up to two years. Sometimes it will do well and then at six months or so start to develop another keloid.

Cryotherapy is popular with some physicians for the treatment of keloids, but we believe that it has the best results on hypertrophic scars, particularly those located on the chest, shoulders, and back.[10] Several moderate-to-hard freezes four to six weeks apart on these postacne scars will flatten them, although the outline of the scar remains, as will its abnormal color and texture.

Radiation therapy can be combined with excision for single keloids and may reduce the incidence of recurrence.[11, 12] Using 1.7 mm of aluminum half-value layer, a one-time-only dose of 500–1,500 roentgens or three alternate-day doses of 300–500 roentgens are adequate. Radiation should be started on the day of or the day following surgery. Appropriate shielding is necessary, and radiation therapy should not be used on keloids on the neck. The dose is dependent on the anatomical site as well as on the size of the keloid. Radiation should be used only by someone well trained and experienced. Another successful treatment for keloids and hypertrophic scars is the application of constant pressure.[13-15] Firm wrapping with a woven elastic bandage, surgically designed straps and corsets, and sometimes even plastic clamps are used. A continuous-pressure clamp on both sides of an ear lobe will help reduce the size of the keloid and help prevent recurrence.[16] This treatment is limited to those areas where pressure can be safely applied for a prolonged period. The most effective results are when the pressure has been in place 12–18 hours per day for several months, and sometimes even up to a year. A custom made Jobst garment will apply pressure over a large area and is said to be helpful for postacne scarring. In our limited experience with this technique, we have had poor results. The garments were uncomfortable and warm, and patients who were not recovering from serious burns were not motivated enough to wear them.

Sometimes it is difficult to assess the results of various treatments obtained by others from reading the literature.[17] Often, the differential between a keloid and a hypertrophic scar is not made carefully. More important, the necessary long-term follow-up sometimes is lacking. It is essential to follow each treatment for several years before any kind of cure rate is assessed.

The African literature describes the systemic administration of methotrexate for extensive and debilitating keloids. Methotrexate is given IM 15–20 mg every four days for two weeks before the keloids are excised and 12.5–15 mg orally or IM every day, three weeks of every four, for six months postoperatively.[18]

REFERENCES

1. Ketchum L.D., Smith J., Robinson D.W., et al.: Treatment of hypertrophic scars, keloids, and scar contracture by triamcinolone acetonide. *Plast. Reconstr. Surg.* 38:209-218, 1966.
2. Murray J.C., Pollack S.V., Pinnel S.R.: Keloids: a review. *J. Am. Acad. Dermatol.* 4:461-470, 1981.
3. Kiil J.C.: Keloids treated with topical injections of triamcinolone acetonide (Kenalog): immediate and long-term results. *Scand. J. Plast. Reconstr. Surg.* 11:169-172, 1977.
4. Maguire H.C.: Treatment of keloids with triamcinolone acetonide injected intralesionally. *J.A.M.A.* 192:325-327, 1965.
5. Griffith B.H., Monroe C.W., McKinney P.: A follow-up study on the treatment of keloids with triamcinolone acetonide. *Plast. Reconstr. Surg.* 46:145-150, 1970.
6. Cosman B., Crikelair G.F., Ju D.M.C., et al.: The surgical treatment of keloids. *Plast. Reconstr. Surg.* 27:335-358, 1961.
7. Griffith B.H.: Treatment of keloids with triamcinolone acetonide. *Plast. Reconstr. Surg.* 38:202–207, 1966.
8. Vallis C.P.: Intralesional injection of keloids and hypertrophic scars with the Dermojet. *Plast. Reconstr. Surg.* 40:255–262, 1967.
9. Ceiley R.I., Babin R.W.: The combined use of cryosurgery and intralesional injections of suspensions of fluorinated adrenocorticosteroids for reducing keloids and hypertrophic scar. *J. Dermatol. Surg. Oncol.* 5:54–56, 1979.
10. Lubritz R.R.: Cryosurgery of benign lesions. *Cutis* 16:426–432, 1975.
11. Levy, D.S., Salter M.M., Roth R.E.: Postoperative irradiation in the prevention of keloids. *Am. J. Roentgenol.* 127:509–510, 1976.
12. Malaker K., Ellis F., Paine C.H.: Keloid scars: a new method of treatment combining surgery with interstitial radiotherapy. *Clin. Radiol.* 27:179–183, 1976.
13. Fujimori R., Hiramoto M., Ofuji S.: Sponge fixation method for treatment of early scars. *Plast. Reconstr. Surg.* 42:322–327, 1968.
14. Brent B.: The role of pressure therapy in management of ear lobe keloids: preliminary report of a controlled study. *Ann. Plast. Surg.* 1:579–581, 1978.

15. Kischer C.W., Shetlar M.R., Shetlar C.L.: Alteration of hypertrophic scars induced by mechanical pressure. *Arch. Dermatol.* 111:60–64, 1975.
16. Snyder G.B.: Button compression for keloids of the lobule. *Br. J. Plast. Surg.* 27:186–187, 1974.
17. Abdel-Fattah A.M.A.: Three distinct varieties of ear lobe keloids in Egypt. *Br. J. Plast. Surg.* 31:261–262, 1978.
18. Onwukwe M.F.: Treating keloids by surgery and methotrexate. *Arch. Dermatol.* 116:158, 1980.

12 / Other Methods of Treating Acne Scarring

EXCISION

Excision of individual acne scars frequently is recommended before dermabrasion or other treatments.

For hypertrophic scars, or scars in which there are acne tunnels and bridges, excision is helpful. For round or oval scars, we prefer the use of other methods listed below. A minimum of one month is recommended before a dermabrasion is done over any of these scar revisions.

Individual sites are anesthetized with 1% Xylocaine with epinephrine 1:100,000. The smallest amount of tissue that just includes the scar, is excised. If the scar can be excised without cutting through the dermis, less gaping will result. We believe the final scar is minimized when there is no gap. There is no reason fibrotic scar tissue cannot be left in place to hold the wound together if adequate normal-appearing tissues can be mobilized and pulled over it. Usually a #11 blade or a Beaver blade gives the most control. Closure is accomplished with 5-0 and 6-0 Prolene. If possible, a buried 6-0 absorbable suture is placed. Through-and-through sutures are removed in five to seven days, and the suture line is splinted with Clearon tapes or similar skin surgical tapes. The patient should be seen in four to five days for reapplication of the tapes to resplint the area. A minimum of two sets of splinting tapes is recommended.

PUNCH GRAFTS—SPONTANEOUSLY HEALING

Removal of a small scar with an Orentreich biopsy punch, followed by spontaneous healing, has been somewhat helpful for depressed acne scars. The end result was a scar that was smaller in diameter and closer to the level of the surface of the skin. Although this method produces smaller scars, it usually leaves scars that are indented and fibrotic. If the patient has depressed and sharp-walled scars 2.0–3.0 mm in diameter, punch removal with secondary healing usually gives a 1.0-mm pit, which may be a sufficient improvement in some cases to make the method worthwhile for the patient. However, we believe that the methods listed below are superior.

PUNCH ELEVATION TECHNIQUE

Norman Orentreich in New York originated this technique in the 1950s, and Cyrus Loo in Hawaii later recommended using thinner-walled punches to gain better cosmetic results. Orentreich uses his own design punches, and Loo has special thin-walled, thick-handled punches made by the Robbins Instrument Company. If the scar is oval, it is stretched on its short axis to form essentially a round scar. Selecting a punch slightly larger than the scar, the punch is inserted through the full thickness of skin. The round cylinder of skin is pulled or snipped free from its fatty attachment. It is replaced or repositioned in the same wound so that the punch graft and the skin surface are on the same plane, even with the surface of the skin. The punch graft is held in place by pressure or with Steri-Strip type of dressings. Occasionally, a punch graft is held in an elevated position with a suture. This technique is best for those scars with smooth, normally pigmented bases.

PUNCH REPLACEMENT TECHNIQUE

In the middle to late 1970s, Orentreich discussed at meetings a revised punch technique in which the punched-out scar was replaced with autogenous skin.

The scars are removed with an Orentreich type punch (Fig 12–1,A). The posterior surface of the ear lobe is anesthetized. If many punches are to be taken, the posterior pinna helical rim and the skin over the mastoid process just posterior to the postauricular sulcus also are good donor sites.

A cylindrical piece of skin and subcutaneous fat cut with a punch 0.5 mm larger than the punch used to remove the scar itself then is taken from the ear area (Fig 12–1,B), and inserted into the hole on the face. Hemostasis on the ear area can be obtained by applying 30% aluminum chloride, Monsel's solution, or Gelfoam plugs and tape. For us it never has been necessary to use hot cautery or electrocoagulation for hemostasis in the ear area.

The cylinder of skin from the ear is placed into the hole in the face and then rotated to where it seems to obtain the best resting position (Fig 12–1,C). For reasons we do not understand, each cylinder has a preferential position, and the only way to find it is to try placing it at various attitudes. It then sits flat with the surface, and the fibrin clot and pressure from the surrounding skin make it stick in surprisingly easily.

The plugs are taped into place with Steri-Strips, Clearon strips, or Op-Site, and the patient is advised to keep the face quiet so that the plugs will stay in place for five to seven days as they heal. If the tapes come loose, we advise the patient to come back immediately so that they can be replaced. We use tape remover to tease up the Steri-Strips gently after five to seven days so that we do not risk pulling the plug out when we take the dressings off. This is an essential part of the treatment because the plugs can be pulled out if much tension is put on them during the first seven to ten days.

The advantages of this technique are two. First, normal skin has replaced a depressed scar. It is amazing how much better a flat defect appears than a depressed scar. Since using this simple technique, we are pleasantly surprised at the number of patients who had a few minimal deep ice-pick type of scars who are significantly improved. In the past we had little sympathy for patients with generally smooth skin who complained of a few defects. After treating their few isolated defects on an otherwise open field of smooth skin, however, we find that their appearance is greatly improved. For patients who wear makeup, the deep ice-pick scar clogs with makeup and will not cover evenly. However, with the punch elevation or punch transplant technique, the makeup goes on smoothly and the blemish is almost entirely hidden. There is a whole new population of patients whom we believe can be benefited.

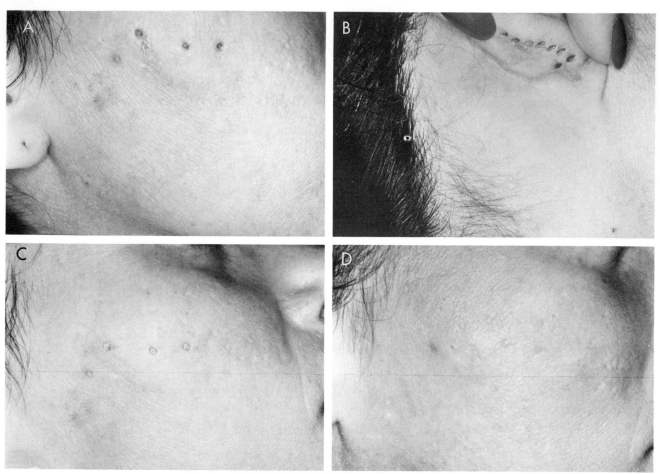

Fig 12–1.—**A,** recipient site scars punched out. **B,** donor sites on the posterior pinna. **C,** transplants in place on the cheek. **D,** four weeks after punch transplants.

Whereas before we were slightly intolerant of their "minimal" problems, now we readily see the need for improvement of these lesions. If the complexion of the face is clear, any little blemish shows; if there are many blemishes, the little defects that we formerly overlooked were not easily seen.

The second major advantage is that the gap that often resulted between the punched out skin and the surrounding skin with the punch elevation technique can be obviated with the punch replacement technique. By using replacement grafts 0.5 mm in diameter larger, there is seldom much visible scar around the graft.

The results of the technique are not perfect (Fig 12–1,D). Patients need to be reminded that they are trading one mark for another. But, in our opinion, the mark that is flush with the surface of the skin is definitely superior to the depressed scar or pit.

Some lesions heal high, and, a month or more later, can be leveled with dermabrasion or with electrocoagulation using the epilating needle and a Bircher hyfrecator set on low current.

To obtain the best results, the largest donor plug from the ear should be no greater than 2.5 mm. When we use donor plugs larger than this, we find that the observing eye picks up the defect and tends to focus on it, whereas smaller defects are quickly passed over.

On thick sebaceous skin, some patients tend to heal with an indentation. Recently we have done a few cases in the following manner. When removing the scar from the thick sebaceous skin, the punch is not cut all the way through the involved skin. Perhaps one-half to three-fourths of the depth of that skin is punched out. Sometimes we do not get all the way to the base of the scar. The scar tissue then is left in the deep dermis, but it holds the dermis together and prevents gaping, which would happen if the dermis is cut through and through. Full-thickness cylinders of postauricular donor skin are taken in the usual manner, 0.5 mm larger than the size of the punch used to cut the defect. These grafts are placed into the facial defect and, obviously, they ride a little high. Sometimes they even heal a little high. However, this provides fresh, nonscarred skin at the surface of the facial defects. These can be leveled with dermabrasion four to six weeks later. In the meantime, while the little plug is riding high, it is surprisingly not unsightly. It does not look much different from a milium or closed comedone. This waiting period is easily accepted by the patients and, after they have undergone dermabrasion, their looks are much improved.

Most recently we have been covering the implanted plugs with strips made from Op-Site. The adhesion is good and the Op-Site appears to give smoother healing of the superficial wound edges, presumably by preventing drying of these edges.

FIBRIN FOAM

We mention this modality for historical interest. It is interesting that Keyes in the original article on the use of the punch in dermatology in 1887 recommended punching out scars and letting them fill in with a clot to produce a better cosmetic result.[1] In the 1960s, injections of fibrin foam by Spangler seemed to produce significant cosmetic benefit.[2] However, the effects were not consistent and the benefit was to only a small percentage of the patients. Modifications of the fibrin foam have been discussed by Sheldon Gottlieb, but the technique, has not gained widespread use.

ZYDERM COLLAGEN

As will become apparent through reading this entire text, most of the time we believe that combined procedures give the best result because acne scarring is not homogeneous, even though from a single disease entity. The advent of Zyderm injectable collagen has been a great boon to the treatment of acne scarring. We have devoted the entirety of chapter 9 to this subject.

REFERENCES

1. Keyes E.L.: The cutaneous punch. *J. Cutan. Genitourin. Dis.* 5:98-1-1, 1887.
2. Spangler A.S.: New treatment of pitted scars, preliminary report. *Arch. Dermatol.* 76:708–711, 1957.
3. Spangler A.S.: Treatment of depressed scars with fibrin form—seventeen years of experience. *J. Dermatol. Surg.* 1:65–69, 1975.

13 / Blepharoplasty

OF ALL THE SURGICAL PROCEDURES discussed in this book, blepharoplasty is the most tedious and demanding. It never should be looked on as a simple procedure, nor should it be conveyed to the patient that it is an easy operation to perform. Whereas the recovery for the patient often is quick and uncomplicated (Plates III and IV, A to C)—far more easy than after a dermabrasion or face peel—the training, skill, and patience needed by the surgeon to perform a blepharoplasty make it an operation that should be entertained only by those fully acquainted with the technique.

It is also an operation that carries considerable risk. Because of those rare cases in which postoperative hemorrhage and infection have led to serious complications, it always is necessary to have justified the risk-vs.-benefit ratio before surgery. This is a procedure in which nothing should be left to chance. The preoperative evaluation and consultation, the actual setting of the surgery, and the scheduling of ample time needed to perform surgery are factors that require careful attention.

PREOPERATIVE EVALUATION

The Patient's Problem

The patient will come in because of baggy eyelids—upper, lower, or both. In the preoperative evaluation, try to discover whether the baggy eyelids are caused by heredity, the normal aging process or premature herniation of fat or are secondary to a medical problem. Detailed analysis will uncover the many components of the patient's problem. Correct preoperative evaluation usually leads to correct surgical planning and design.

Three separate tissues most commonly contribute to the appearance of the baggy eye. There can be excess and redundant skin, hypertrophic orbicularis oculi muscle, or protuberant or herniated fat from the fat pockets of both the upper and lower eyelids. The design of the operation will be contingent on which of those tissues needs to be altered. Not only does the design of the operation vary with each patient but it may vary between the eyes of each patient.

During the preoperative evaluation, observe the patient in the sitting position and encourage the patient to talk, laugh, squint, and move the eyes upward, sideways, and downward. While you are observing, take note of the movement of the eyelids, the bulging of the orbicularis oculi muscle, and the bulging of the protuberant fat pad. The fat pads can also be checked by gentle pressure on the globe. While the patient lightly closes his eyes, press gently on the globe through the upper eyelid. The lower fat pads bulge and can be evaluated for needed excision.

There is no substitute for the time spent talking with the patient and critically examining all of these factors. The patient should have a mirror in hand during this interview so that you can call attention to your findings. The patient needs to realize the full extent of the problem and all factors that contribute to the appearance of the eyes.

During the same examination using the mirror, you will discover what the patient desires to accomplish. A moderate bulging of the orbicularis oculi when the patient squints or laughs often is the sign of a youthful eye. The patient should be encouraged to understand that this is not abnormal whereas a large bulging can be trimmed and the appearance improved. Differentiation should be made between the bagginess of protruding fat pads and eyelid edema, which usually is not corrected by surgery. The fat pads of the upper cheeks over the malar prominence also will not be affected by blepharoplasty.

The next observation is of the skin of the eyelid itself. Only the color and texture of the skin may be bothering the patient, in which case a blepharoplasty is not indicated. For finely wrinkled skin that is not redundant, a peel would be more effective. Skin that is sun-damaged would respond to peeling. The eyelids should be examined for benign lesions and these, too, should be discussed and possibly treated prior to or during the blepharoplasty. The patient must be made aware of these lesions' presence and must give permission for removal. Milia, epidermal cysts, sebaceous hyperplasias, xanthomas, elastoses, giant comedones, and syringoma are common around the eyes. The numbers and sizes of these lesions will affect the planning of the surgery.

A history of intermittent swelling related to the hormonal cycles commonly is found in females. The patient must understand that this type of edema will not be improved. A history of recurrent allergies that manifest as conjunctivitis and swelling of the eyes also may affect the final cosmetic appearance, since the same problems will continue after the surgery.

The elasticity of the lower lids must be examined carefully in any patient over 55 years of age. The lid may become lax, which not only contributes to the appearance of baggy eyes but also increases the incidence of postoperative lateral scleral show (the amount of white sclera showing between the upper margin of the lower lid and the edge of the iris) or true ectropion. The strength of the lower lid can be tested by picking it up between the thumb and forefinger, pulling it 1.0 or 2.0 mm from the globe and watching how fast it snaps back. The normal lower lid will snap back quickly whereas one that is lax may stay bulged and only slowly return to its position in contact with the globe. The lax lower lid can be repaired at the time of blepharoplasty, but if this is not noticed preoperatively, postoperative complications are more likely.

The lateral upper eyelid just below the orbital rim must be examined for the lacrimal gland. Rarely, the lacrimal gland is ptotic or hypertrophied. There is no reason why the gland cannot be sutured back to its normal position or trimmed during the time of surgery, but if this is not found prior to surgery, the final result will not be as good as it could have been.

Sometimes asymmetry is found. The patient must be examined carefully for asymmetry of the palpebral fissures, the position of the eye within the bony orbit, the amount of overhang of redundant upper eyelid tissue, the position of the eyebrows, and the amount of sclera showing on each side. The asymmetries often can be corrected during the procedure, but they must be discovered prior to the operation. The patient must be made aware of the preexisting asymmetry and know that the surgery cannot guarantee perfect symmetry afterward. We often tell patients that we will try to correct it but that a second procedure may be necessary to try to correct further asymmetries that might develop. *The asymmetry before surgery should be documented on the chart and with photographs.*

Observe the eyebrow and its location with regard to the upper lid. The problem may be ptotic eyebrow as well as baggy eyelids. Many times a patient, particularly a male, will need an eyebrow lift in conjunction with or instead of blepharoplasty. The eyebrow lift should be done prior to blepharoplasty. By demonstrating the looseness of the eyebrow, particularly on the lateral one-half, the patient will realize that blepharoplasty will take out the redundant eyelid skin but not correct the hooding from a ptotic lateral eyebrow.

Usually the distance between the eyebrow and the eyelid is smaller in men than in women. This must be discussed with male patients so that they do not have the mistaken idea that eyelid surgery is going to give the appearance of much wider eyes—although the eyes can be made to look wider with certain techniques, which will be discussed below. The patient's exact desires should be understood and discussed.

Baseline Ophthalmologic Examination

It is essential that all blepharoplasty patients have a complete ophthalmologic examination. We insist that the report from the ophthalmologist be on the chart before the patient can be scheduled for operation. If we know the ophthalmologist whom the patient plans to see, we request a preblepharoplasty examination. However, if we do not know the ophthalmologist, we send along a specific list of items that we want examined. We ask for visual acuity, examination of the muscles of extraocular motion, the visual fields, pressures, slit-lamp examination of the cornea and lens, funduscopy, a measured test for tear production, and evaluation for ptosis and blepharoptosis.

Blepharoptosis is something that the surgeon himself can and should try to evaluate. However, having the ophthalmologist "check you" on the existence of preoperative blepharoptosis is helpful. If blepharoptosis is present, the etiology should be sought and the operation designed to help correct the blepharoptosis, if possible. Several procedures for the correction of blepharoptosis not discussed in this chapter could become part of the physician's surgical skills should he elect to train in these additional procedures. Otherwise, patients who have severe or obvious blepharoptosis should not have blepharoplasty or should have it done by a properly trained surgeon.

The ophthalmologist can also help in the medical evaluation of the patient for thyroid disease, renal disease, hereditary edema, diabetes, etc. Any of these conditions can affect the final outcome of the procedure and should be noted ahead of time.

The Patient's Goals

The patient may come to you asking about baggy eyelids, but the entire aging face should be considered briefly. If the eyelids are prematurely aging or show hereditary changes that make them look baggy, a blepharoplasty alone may be adequate. If the eyelids are only part of many changes of aging, repair of the eyelids may give the patient a false sense of improved appearance. The cosmetic surgeon must point out that the eyelid changes may be one of several areas that could use improving and that the blepharoplasty might be only one of a series of operations that the patient should consider.

The design of the operation will be affected by the patient's goals. The patient may want to change premature aging of the eyes so that they will look normal for their age. This calls for much more conservative surgery that does not alter the size or shape of the palpebral fissure or the distance of the upper eyelid between the eyelash line and the supratarsal crease. On the other hand, the patient may want to regain as much beauty and attractiveness as possible. For this patient, more attention can be given to increasing the amount of upper lid show between the lash line and the supratarsal crease and consideration of additional procedures, such as eyebrow lifts and face peels.

The patient may be interested only in the functional problems of eye fatigue from the heavy redundancy of the upper lids or correction of the loss of upper lateral gaze due to overhanging upper lids.

Also, some cosmetic problems are significant, such as the inability to wear eyelid makeup because of the smearing and folding of the redundant upper lids, the problem of the dissipated appearance of the young patient who has a hereditary herniation of fat pads, and the tired and unkempt look of the patient who has dark rings and shadows secondary to redundant skin or herniations of the fat of the lower lids.

The patient must be told about results of the procedure that are unobtainable. Sometimes the patient expects a blepharoplasty to correct the crow's-feet and, of course, this will not happen. Face peeling, dermabrasion, and some modified face-lifts may temporarily improve the crow's-feet. The crepe-paper skin of the lids also is not altered with blepharoplasty alone. Peeling at a later date can help correct this as well as pigmentary problems of the lids. The puffy cheek pouches over the malar prominences are in no way altered by blepharoplasty and actually may be accentuated if the eyelid redundancy and puffiness have been corrected by the procedure.

Preoperative Instructions

Before the day of surgery, we give the patient a list of all postoperative instructions. This allows the patient to plan for the care that will be needed in the immediate postoperative phase and to obtain the necessary supplies. Often, if these instructions are given before the day of surgery or even sent home in a printed form to the patient before surgery, his comprehension is greatly improved and thus, compliance is more likely. We have our postoperative instructions printed and given to the patient before the operation.

Once the procedure has been designed and scheduled, we preview with the patient specific preoperative instructions. We ask that the face be washed the night before and the morning of surgery with Hibiclens, which we provide. Instructions are given not to wear makeup or tight-fitting clothing the day of surgery. Since our operation is done with only local anesthesia, we ask that a normal light breakfast or lunch (whichever is appropriate) be eaten prior to coming to the office. It is important for the patient to be accompanied by someone who can drive him home after the surgery. We do not want the blepharoplasty patient to go home in a taxi unattended or in any conveyance other than a private automobile. Also, we ask that arrangements be made to have someone stay with the patient for the first 24 hours—someone who can make a phone call if there are postoperative complications and who is responsible enough to recognize problems and know how to get in touch with the physician.

UPPER LID TECHNIQUE

Marking

The skin to be excised from the upper lid should be marked with the patient in the sitting position and before the injection of anesthesia. We use a gentian violet pencil that is sterile and disposable, but this is not ideal. As the patient blinks, particularly if the skin is redundant, the lines tend to smear. Other physicians use brilliant green and a sharpened wooden applicator stick.

Some physicians grasp the skin of the upper eyelid with the specially designed Green Fixation Forceps, which allows them to pick up a greater amount of redundant skin and make the markings. Some physicians recommend injecting hyaluronidase prior to marking. The skin becomes doughy and, when pinched up, the skin stays elevated long enough to complete exact marking.

Anesthesia

We do all blepharoplasties with local anesthesia. Since we always do the uppers first, we inject the uppers first and then the lowers with 1% Xylocaine with epinephrine 1:100,000, using a 30-gauge, 1-in. needle. We start with the lateral canthal markings and inject under the entire upper eyelid skin using 1.5–2.0 ml, first on the right and then on the left. At this time we also estimate where the middle and medial fat pockets are and inject about 0.1–0.2 ml into these pockets. Some physicians will wait until just before these pockets are opened before injecting local anesthesia.

We wait 10–15 minutes to allow for the diffusion of the Xylocaine and the onset of vasoconstriction.

Patients tolerate local anesthesia extremely well. We talk to them throughout the injection and point out that their discomfort will last only a few seconds. This avoids the risk of nausea, the postdrug feelings of sedatives and systemic analgesics, and makes it easier for them to leave the operating room quicker. Local anesthetic enables the patient to follow instructions to look up, open his eyes, etc. We have not had any patients ever disagree with the approach of simple local anesthesia only.

Design

The most common shape of redundant skin to be removed from the upper eyelid is that of a simple ellipse (Fig 13–1). The ellipse is made wider at the lateral one-third of the upper lid. There usually is more redundancy of skin in this area, and the laxity of the skin over the lateral eyebrow and the temple causes a quicker return of the lateral hooding. The ellipse starts just over the punctum on the medial side and extends to a line just above the lateral canthus if the blepharoplasty is done primarily to remove fat or redundant upper-lid skin.

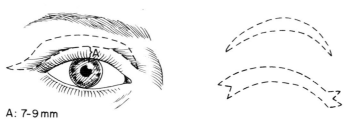

A: 7-9 mm

Fig 13–1.—Extent and position of incisions for removal of
redundant skin in upper eyelid.

If there are prominent crow's-feet and the skin at the lateral edge of the eye
and the lateral orbit is redundant, the ellipse is carried into one of the crow's-
feet. The extension into the crow's-feet area should be at least on a horizontal
line or in a slightly superior line. The extension onto the crow's-feet area
should be above a line extended horizontally from the commissure of the lateral canthus. Since lower-lid blepharoplasties often are performed at the same
time, there is a tendency for this portion of the suture line to be pulled lower
than desired. Sometimes the complication of a lateral canthal fold develops if
this incision is carried too far inferiorly.

The placement of the inferior limb of this ellipse is most important. The
literature states that the lower line of the incision at the level of the midpupillary line should be between 7.0 and 9.0 mm above the ciliary margin. It is
important to measure this distance with the patient sitting. Just how much
above the ciliary margin the line should be placed depends on the patient's
natural supratarsal crease. For example, in men it generally is lower than in
women; in Orientals it is lower than in Occidentals. If one were to make the
lower margin of the incision at the full 9.0 mm above the ciliary margin on an
Oriental patient, it should be done only after the physician and the patient
have agreed that they are trying to achieve a more rounded or Western eye.
For women who are trying to achieve an eye that is more open and more
amenable to the use of makeup, some physicians will make the supratarsal
crease at the full 9.0 mm from the ciliary margin.

The location of the upper edge of the incision is based on the amount of
redundant skin that must be removed. As mentioned above, this line can be
determined by pinching the skin and estimating how much redundant skin
needs to be excised. It is important to differentiate between eyelid skin and
non-eyelid skin, which is inferior to the eyebrows. The redundancy can be
taken out only from eyelid skin, and one should not make the mistake of
pulling non-eyelid skin into the supratarsal crease, since it usually is more
sebaceous, thicker, and a slightly different color. Such an error would result
in a thickened and unsightly eyelid, with the possibility of functional problems.

A variation on the cutting of the upper limb of this excision involves first
cutting the lower limb, undermining the remainder of the upper eyelid superior to that incision, and then pulling the redundant upper-eyelid skin over the
lower incision to measure that redundancy before it is excised (Fig 13–2). The
resultant dog-ears at each end are repaired in standard fashion. This technique
theoretically and in practice tends to reduce the incidence of excessive removal
of skin. However, we have not believed that the extra effort for this technique

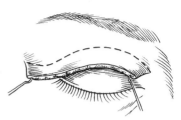

Fig 13–2.—Variation of technique in which the lower limb of the excision is cut first and the redundancy measured before the upper incision is made.

is necessary if the physician is careful and conservative in his preoperative markings.

There are designs for the redundant skin of the upper eyelid other than the simple ellipse (see Fig 13–1). Lewis[1] in 1969 proposed that the lateral end of the ellipse be designed as a Z-plasty, with the skin at the extension of the lateral canthus. The idea was to turn the skin at the lateral canthus more superiorly to avoid the lateral canthal fold or the drooping lateral canthus that sometimes may result. Webster and others in 1978 discussed the use of an M-plasty at each end of the ellipse.[2, 3] This allowed more tissue to be removed above the medial puncta without extending the excision medial to the puncta and creating the risk of a medial canthal fold or scar. The lateral M-plasty was designed to move tissue of the lateral canthus in a superior and lateral fashion as opposed to the standard technique, which basically moved the redundant skin of the lateral eyelid that was lateral to the canthus in an inferior fashion. This technique has a great deal of merit and in specific cases would be the design of choice.

Excision

The patient is placed in a comfortable supine position, the anesthesia given, and, after an appropriate wait, the skin of the upper lid is excised. We cut exactly on our inferior line and always cut just inside our superior line, giving us a built-in conservative approach and a safety factor. The skin is dissected with small iris scissors from the underlying stroma and orbicularis oculi muscle. The excised skin is placed on a cotton sponge, moistened with normal saline in a sterile Petri dish, sealed, marked, and placed in the refrigerator for 24 hours in case a graft might be needed to repair excess skin removal from the lower eyelids.

Hemostasis then is obtained. We use a Bircher hyfrecator—monopolar—with settings fairly low. We believe that with the use of the hyfrecator and cotton-tipped applicators we can control the bleeding better than with any other instrument we have used. We have tried bipolar current and fine forceps attached to various machines and have not found anything as simple and as effective as the simple Bircher hyfrecator. The secret to making the Bircher hyfrecator work for hemostasis is to have good control of the bleeding into the field so that there is essentially no blood escaping onto the area being desiccated.

Next, cut a 1.0–2.0-mm-wide strip of orbicularis oculi muscle the entire width of the eyelid (Fig 13–3). Start above the lateral canthus just superior to the superior edge of the tarsal plate and cut the strip to just above the puncta. By lifting up the muscle gently with a small-toothed forceps, such as Bishop

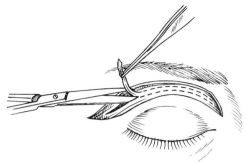

Fig 13–3.—Excision of a strip of orbicularis oculi muscle the width of the eyelid.

Harmon, we have good control of the excision and cut only muscle without fear of cutting underlying tissues. Occasionally, some hemostasis is needed after the muscle is cut.

The whitish, firm orbital septum then is visible and opened either by stab wounds and spreading with the iris scissors or with actual scissor or knife incision along its length.

Lipectomy

Not all upper-lid blepharoplasties require lipectomy. There are some cases, particularly in the elderly, in which only the redundant skin needs to be removed. However, most of the time, the patients can benefit both functionally and cosmetically by removal of excessive or protuberant periorbital fat. Some surgeons believe that a strip of periorbital fat should be taken from the entire width of the eye to make the supratarsal sulcus more even and prominent. Others believe that only a little bit from the middle and most of the excess medial protuberant fat should be removed. We try to adjust this on an individual patient basis. Good preoperative analysis of the patient helps us decide. However, the amount of fat that easily protrudes once the orbital septum is opened is the best guide for the amount of fat to remove (Fig 13–4,A).

The fat is handled most delicately. We use a small-toothed forceps in one hand and a cotton-tipped applicator in the other (Fig 13–4,B), gently teasing the orbital fat from its pocket through the incised orbital septum. The fat of the lateral middle pocket is yellow and stringy whereas the fat from the medial middle pocket is more ivory-colored and firm.

We always use the technique of clamping the fat with a small, straight mosquito hemostat, using the scalpel or scissors to cut off the fat protruding from the hemostat (Fig 13–4,C), desiccating the fat while it is in the hemostat, and then releasing the clamp (Fig 13–4,D). This may be an excessive maneuver for the upper eyelids, since there is less incidence of bleeding and less chance of retrobulbar hematoma. However, we like the habit of being careful with the fat and believe that the extra effort is well worth the peace of mind and relative safety. Only rarely is there a bleeder that is not controlled in this fashion, and, occasionally, a 6-0 Vicryl or Dexon suture is needed. Some surgeons place a figure eight suture behind the clamp for additional security.

It must be emphasized that this fat must not be tugged on or handled roughly and that only the amount of fat that protrudes easily should be ex-

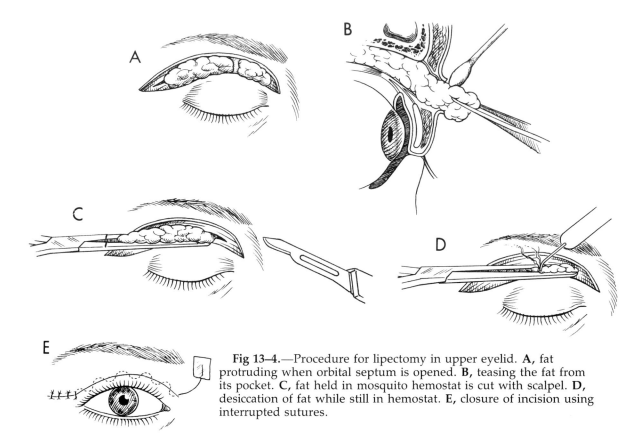

Fig 13–4.—Procedure for lipectomy in upper eyelid. **A,** fat protruding when orbital septum is opened. **B,** teasing the fat from its pocket. **C,** fat held in mosquito hemostat is cut with scalpel. **D,** desiccation of fat while still in hemostat. **E,** closure of incision using interrupted sutures.

cised. Tugging on the fat may tear blood vessels deeper in the orbit and result in undetected bleeding.

At this point, we tease the edges of the incision together and move to the contralateral eye. Then we carry out the same surgery to the same point on the second eye. This maneuver allows us an extra 15 minutes of observation of an open wound before closure to be sure that there are no delayed or overlooked bleeders.

Closure

We return to the first eye, tease open the incision, and carefully inspect for any bleeders. Also, at this time, we inspect to see if there is any more fat that easily protrudes. The wound in the orbital septum again is teased together.

The orbital septum and the muscle are not sutured. The skin is teased side to side, and any irregular edges, redundancies, or dog-ears, are excised at this time.

The closure is made with 6-0 nylon, Prolene, Ethibond, or Ethiflex sutures (Fig 13–4,E). In the area of the crow's-feet, we use interrupted sutures and across the eyelid a running subcuticular suture. The running subcuticular technique works beautifully in this area, since the skin is under little or no tension. It is important to bring a loop of suture over the surface of the incision lines at about the midpupillary line. This facilitates suture removal. Start laterally and suture medially. A small knot or loop can be left at the medial end or the suture can be continued under the skin, brought out on the lateral side of the nose, and simply taped on the glabella. This latter technique allows the suture to adjust when the eyes start to move and is less likely to produce puckers or wrinkles. It also is less likely to produce a small pustule at the knot site, which later may leave a small, unsightly scar.

The first eye is closed and the second eye is inspected again and closed in a like manner.

A light coat of Bacitracin or similar ointment is placed over the incision lines, and no dressings are used. If we are going to proceed with the lower-lid blepharoplasty, we recess at this time and allow the patient to relax on the table. This little break makes the entire procedure more pleasant and more enjoyable for all involved.

LOWER LID TECHNIQUE

Anesthesia

The anesthesia again is with 1% Xylocaine with epinephrine 1:100,000. It is injected through a 30-gauge, 1-in. needle starting at the lateral canthal edge and extending under the lower ciliary margin to the medial puncta. The middle and medial fat pockets also are infiltrated with 0.1–0.2 ml of local anesthesia. If undermining is anticipated down to the level of the bony orbital margin, this area also is infiltrated.

The Incision

The incision is made with the scalpel or started with the scalpel and continued with scissors, 1.0–2.0 mm below the lower ciliary margin (Fig 13–5,A). The extension onto the crow's-feet area should be made with an acute angle inferiorly. Some physicians recommend that it be made horizontally. When both upper and lower blepharoplasties are performed, leave a minimum of 5.0 mm between the lateral extensions of the incisions. It is better to leave 8.0 mm to help prevent any contracture and lateral epicanthal fold formation.

There can be a great deal of variation from this point on with the lower-lid blepharoplasty.[4–6] The preoperative analysis as to which problems need correction will indicate which technique should be used. The amount of redundant skin, the herniation of the fat, the laxity of the orbicularis oculi muscle, and the elasticity of the lower lid are the key factors. Some physicians almost always use a skin muscle flap if the main problem is herniation or excessive fat with little skin to be removed. If the problem is mostly one of redundant skin without much herniation of fat, only a skin flap is created. If the lower lid is so lax that a wedge excision will be necessary, a skin flap is created, with dissection of the muscle as needed. Keep in mind, scar formation between the skin and muscle in some cases may have led to scleral show or hound dog eyes or true ectropion even in cases in which no, or not much, skin was removed.

Our technique is to incise the skin with a scalpel just below the lash line. If the patient has mostly herniation of fat and not much redundant skin, we use

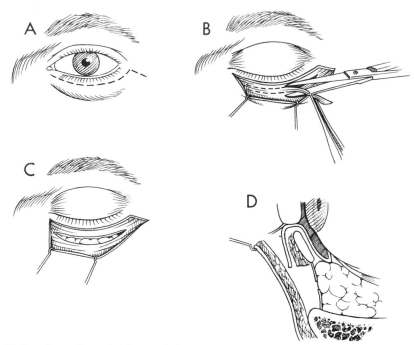

Fig 13–5.—Procedure for lower lid. **A,** incision is made 1.0–2.0 mm below lower ciliary border. **B,** excision of 2.0-mm strip of orbicularis oculi muscle. **C,** incision of orbital septum permits fat to protrude. **D,** skin-muscle flap reduces problem of postoperative scar formation.

the scissors to dissect the skin from the orbicularis oculi muscle for only 5.0–6.0 mm inferior to the incision line. We then excise a 2.0-mm strip of orbicularis oculi muscle approximately 3.0–4.0 mm inferior to the skin incision (Fig 13–5,B). The orbital septum is then exposed, incised carefully, and the redundant fat protrudes (Fig 13–5,C).

Inferior to the strip where the muscle was removed and the septum incised, the lid acts as a skin muscle flap. After the redundant fat has been excised, the entire flap is draped over the eyelid, the flap is a skin only flap where it was dissected free from the muscle, and is a skin muscle flap inferior to that. The entire combined flap is then pulled superiorly and laterally and draped over the lower eyelid area. We prefer this technique because there is a limited amount of dissection of skin from the underlying muscle. The resulting scar formation between skin and muscle that was dissected sometimes causes problems with the downward pull on the lower eyelid, leading to the hound dog eye.

If the patient has massively redundant skin, the skin must be undermined to the level of the orbital rim. Then the muscle strip is removed, and the procedure is the same as when only 4.0–5.0 mm of skin is undermined for those cases in which not redundancy but herniated fat is the problem (Fig 13–5,D). Hemostasis then is obtained in the same fashion as for the upper eyelids.

Lipectomy

In the lower eyelids, most of the excess fat is in the middle fat compartment. Occasionally, some of the medial fat is removed. More commonly, a small

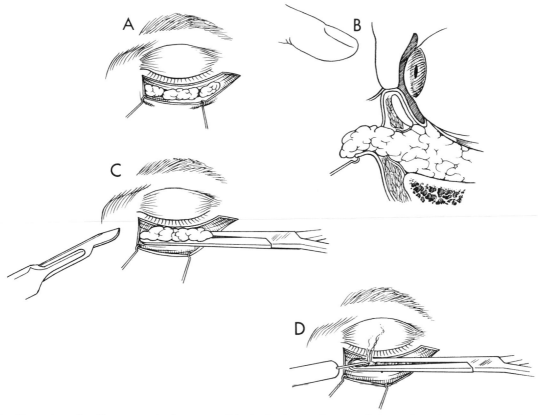

Fig 13–6.—Procedure for lipectomy in lower eyelid. **A,** fat is gently teased through stab wounds in the orbital septum. **B,** only that fat which protrudes naturally or with gentle pressure should be removed. **C,** fat is held in mosquito hemostat and cut. **D,** fat is desiccated while still in hemostat.

amount is removed from the lateral fat pocket. It is important not to remove too much from the lateral pocket, since this can create an unsightly hollowness at the lateral edge of the eye.

The technique for teasing the fat gently through the stab wounds in the orbital septum is the same as for the upper eyelid (Fig 13–6,A). Only the amount of fat that protrudes naturally or can be made to protrude by gentle pressure on the globe should be excised (Fig 13–6,B). Hemostasis is much more important in this area than in the upper eyelid. As before, we clamp all fat (Fig 13–6,C), cut it, desiccate it while it is in the clamp (Fig 13–6,D), release the clamp, and inspect for any bleeders. Only occasionally are suture ligatures or figure eights necessary.

At this point, we drape the skin over the wound of this eye and go to the contralateral eye and carry the surgery to the same stage.

Muscle Suspension

If there is a great deal of laxity in the lower eyelid, sometimes it is helpful to suspend the lateral edge of the orbicularis oculi to the periosteum or fascia over the lateral portion of the orbit (Fig 13–7).[7, 8] Often, the lateral portions of the orbicularis oculi fibers are atrophic and widely dispersed. It is not difficult to

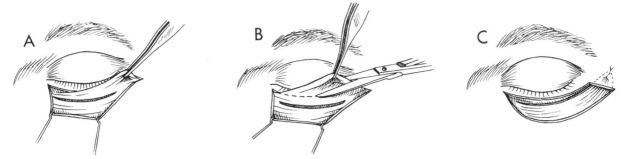

Fig 13–7.—Muscle suspension technique to improve appearance when there is laxity in the lower eyelid. **A,** examination for excessive muscle. **B,** removal of excess muscle. **C,** suturing to lateral orbital periosteum or fascia.

place a small permanent suture to elevate this muscle to the lateral orbital periosteum or fascia. If the muscle is not atrophic but simply lax, it can be imbricated (folded on itself) with a small permanent suture. Suspension may pull the muscle or the skin-muscle flap superiorly enough that there is excessive muscle, which requires trimming.

If any type of suspension technique is undertaken, extreme care must be used not to create a bulge or crease at the lower lateral canthal area or to create an asymmetry by elevating or tensing one muscle more than the other. This muscle suspension technique greatly reduces the incidence of scleral show (that increased amount of sclera seen below the iris and the lower lid), or ectropion and also helps to smooth the skin of the lower-lid blepharoplasty.

Skin Excision

Having carried the operation to the point of fat removal or muscle suspension in both eyes, we return to the first eye and open the wound to inspect for late-developing bleeders. The septum, skin, and muscle are aligned and the skin is carefully teased into position with instruments or moistened, cotton-

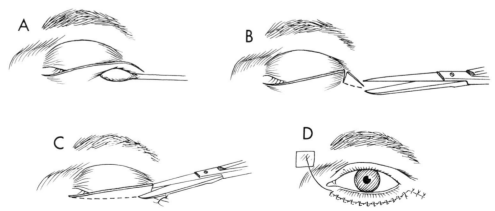

Fig 13–8.—Closure of lower eyelid. **A,** skin teased into smooth approximation with a cotton-tipped applicator. **B,** wedge of excess skin taken lateral to the lateral canthus may be all the skin that needs to be removed. **C,** removal of triangle of skin. **D,** closure with a simple running suture, lateral to medial.

tipped applicators (Fig 13–8,A), with smooth approximation over the orbital septum. The skin is draped in a superior and lateral fashion rather than strictly superior. Once the eyelid is draped into place, we ask the patient to look upward and open the mouth. This puts the most stress on the lower eyelid and gives us a guide as to how much skin is needed to completely cover the lower eyelid at its most extreme point of tension.

In many patients, a wedge of excess skin taken lateral to the lateral canthus is all the skin that needs to be removed (Fig 13–8,B). It is important to be extremely conservative in removing any skin of the lower eyelid parallel to the lid margin between the midpupillary line and the punctum. In cases of marked redundancy of skin, 1.0–2.0 mm of excess skin may need to be removed between the lateral canthus and the midpupillary line. Rarely is it necessary to remove more than 1.0 mm of skin between the midpupillary line and the medial punctum. In many cases, no skin parallel to the lid margin is removed.

The design of the triangle of skin to be removed at the lateral canthus depends on the initial incision and on the skin redundancy. This can be determined only after it has been undermined and draped over the lower eyelid (Fig 13–8,C).

We usually excise the lateral wedge of excess skin and place one to two interrupted key sutures lateral to the lateral canthus. The patient again is asked to gaze upward and open the mouth. At this time, we conservatively remove any more tissue as necessary.

Closure

The lower lid is closed with 6-0 nylon, Prolene, Ethibond, or Ethiflex with a subcuticular running or a simply running suture (Fig 13–8,D). Again, we suture from lateral to medial and, at the medial margin, the needle is slipped under the skin to the lateral edge of the nose, brought to the surface, and taped on the glabella.

No dressings are necessary. The suture line is covered with Bacitracin ointment.

POSTOPERATIVE CARE

Usually at about the time the procedure is finished, all the local anesthesia has worn off and the patient experiences mild-to-moderate discomfort at the incision lines. We give the patient Tylenol with codeine in the office and have him take the first dose before leaving. Instructions are also given to remain at bed rest with the head slightly elevated and to use lightweight ice bags over both eyes intermittently for the rest of the day of surgery.

Sometimes there is slight inability to completely close the upper eyelids. If we have any doubts about the patient's ability to protect the cornea, instructions and materials are given so that the eyes may be patched shut during the first postoperative night.

We also give instructions to not watch television or read for the first 24 hours and to keep the use of the eyes to a minimum for the next two or three days.

Careful instructions also are given about the need to call the physician if there is a sudden onset of pain, swelling, or formation of a black-and-blue appearance around the eyes. A little oozing from the suture line is considered normal, but we carefully warn the patient to call us and come in if any other side effects develop.

We instruct the patient to clean the suture lines gently with hydrogen peroxide and cotton-tipped applicators for the first several days after surgery, and then cover the incision lines with Bacitracin ointment. The patient is also told to refrain from any strenuous activity until seen again in the office. We remove the sutures after four or five days.

The patient is advised that ecchymoses may be moderate or severe and may last for up to two to two and one-half weeks. Wide sunglasses help not only for camouflage but also help to keep the patient from squinting, reducing movement and tension on the suture line.

COMPLICATIONS

Hematomas

If a large hematoma develops during the first 24 hours postoperatively, it is best to take out the sutures, take down the incision, and search for the bleeder. At that time, hemostasis can be obtained with electrocoagulation or with a suture ligature. If a large asymptomatic hematoma develops after the fourth or fifth day, it can be left for ten to twelve days and then drained through a small stab wound or incision along the suture line at one end or the other. Sometimes when large hematomas organize there is a liquefactive phase during which they can be evacuated by a large needle.

Small asymptomatic hematomas developing early or late can be left to resolve on their own. They often create a bluish discolored subcutaneous nodule that can persist for several months but eventually resolves with no permanent mark. The patient needs much support during this time. If a hematoma is associated with an alteration in vision, it must be evacuated immediately.

Visual Changes Postblepharoplasty

If excessive swelling or a hematoma occurs, vision should be checked closely and monitored, since unilateral or bilateral loss of vision would be a most grievous complication. The visual acuity can be checked with the preoperative visual acuity on record.

If there is visual loss, the retina should be examined and careful attention paid to the retinal artery and vein for signs of occlusion. The wound should be taken down immediately and any blood clots removed to reduce pressure on these vessels. Emergency consultation with a surgical ophthalmologist is recommended.

Prominent or Unsightly Scarring

Time is the best treatment for a persistent erythematous scar or slightly hypertrophic scar. Makeup also is helpful on the female patient. Occasionally, scars can be injected with triamcinolone acetonide, 4–20 mg/ml. However, it is difficult to inject the medicine into the small linear scars alone without getting it into the surrounding tissues.

Suture Tracks

Often the suture tracks show on the upper eyelids if the subcuticular sutures were too large or were left in too long. Many of these will resolve on their own, but they can be marsupialized by slipping a hook or one side of a small set of iris scissors under the suture track and incising across the top. This lays the track open, and it reepithelializes completely, usually with little residual scarring.

Scleral Show or Ectropion on the Lower Lid

Scleral show may develop on the lower eyelid even though the surgery was performed carefully and properly. The present-day theory is that if a skin flap was used there is scar contraction between the skin flap and the muscle, which leads to foreshortening and thus to pulling on the lateral edge of the lower eyelid. If there is gross scar contracture or too much skin was removed from the lower eyelid, ectropion can occur. Mild ectropion can be corrected by frequent upward massage of the lower eyelids and time. More severe ectropion will require lateral canthoplasty or even a full-thickness skin graft. The graft donor site can be the retroauricular skin or any remaining redundant upper-eyelid skin.

Webbing of the Medial Canthus

This usually is the result of extending the excision for the upper lid too far medially. A small Z-plasty over the webbed portion of the upper eyelid or several small Z-plasties often are helpful in resolving this complication.

Blepharoptosis—Dropping of the Upper Eyelid

Blepharoptosis often is the result of damage to the levator aponeurosis during the surgery. This can result more easily if fat was removed from the lateral fat pocket. The levator aponeurosis lies close to the surface if there is not a great deal of fat in the lateral pocket. The blepharoptosis may be temporary and can be common the first few days after surgery if there was any fixation of the aponeurosis during the surgery. Most of the time, this problem will resolve spontaneously within several months. However, if it does not, a second operation is necessary to resect any scar contracture or to repair the levator aponeurosis.

Sometimes blepharoptosis was not recognized prior to surgery, in which case it can be confusing and frustrating for both the physician and the patient.

Misplacement of the Eyelid Crease

Despite careful marking and careful surgery, at the completion of the operation the physician may find marked asymmetry between the placement of the supratarsal eyelid crease on the upper lids. If this is the case, the offending side should be taken down and corrected immediately. More commonly, however, the crease is placed too low because the surgeon tried to resect too much skin and stretch the more superior eyelid skin too far. In these cases, it would have been better to have a levator aponeurosis fixation in conjunction with the blepharoplasty.

If the patient is unhappy with the location of the supratarsal crease, at least have the satisfaction of knowing that you measured the location of that crease prior to surgery and can assure the patient that it is within the limits of the recommended distance from the ciliary margin. Patients may not be happy with this answer, but it is less likely that they will pursue any further action.

Asymmetry

Even though asymmetry was recognized prior to surgery and attempts were made to re-create symmetry, occasionally it is everyone's misfortune to discover a few days after surgery that there is asymmetry that is obvious. We try to discuss this possibility with the patient prior to surgery and tell the patient that if a further "tuck up" or pucker removal is needed at a later date, this is to be considered part of the original surgery. Usually the patient is not unhappy if this happens and will willingly come back in a few weeks for a minor adjustment.

Lagophthalmos—Failure of the Upper Lid to Close Completely

There naturally is some lagophthalmos with the standard upper-eyelid blepharoplasty. For this reason, the patient is instructed to be sure that the eyelids cover the cornea the first night after surgery. However, if lagophthalmos persists for several days, it may be that too much skin was removed from the upper lids. Often, as all of the edema settles out, the eyelids will close completely. However, if the lagophthalmos is marked, a secondary surgical repair may be necessary to graft in more skin or to release orbital septum, which may have been incorporated into the closure of the skin.

REFERENCES

1. Lewis J.R.: The Z-blepharoplasty. *Plast. Reconstr. Surg.* 44:331-335, 1969.
2. Webster R.C., Smith R.C., Davidson T.M., et al.: A flap suspension technique in blepharoplasty on lower lids. *J. Dermatol. Surg. Oncol.* 2:159-165, 1978.
3. Courtiss E.H., Webster R.C., White M.F.: Use of double W-plasty in upper blepharoplasty. *Plast. Reconstr. Surg.* 53:25-28, 1974.
4. Klatsky S.A., Manson P.N.: Separate skin and muscle flaps in lower-lid blepharoplasty. *Plast. Reconstr. Surg.* 2:151-156, 1981.
5. Owsley J.W., Jr.: Blepharoplasty variations, in Goulian D., Courtiss E.H. (eds.): *Symposium on Surgery of the Aging Face,* vol. 19, St. Louis, C.V. Mosby, 1978, chap. 17, pp. 163-170.
6. Kostianovsky A.S.: Modification of the cutaneous muscular flap approach for lower blepharoplasty. *Aesth. Plast. Surg.* 3:153, 1979.
7. Mladick R.A.: Muscle suspension lower blepharoplasty. *Plast. Reconstr. Surg.* 64:171, 1979.
8. Foerster D.W.: A new method for tightening the orbicularis oculi muscles in blepharoplasty. *Aesth. Plast. Surg.* 3:265, 1979.

14 / A Basic Face-lift

RALPH LUIKART II, M.D.*

RHYTIDOSIS means wrinkle and "ectomy" means excision; hence, the term rhytidectomy for a face-lift is a misnomer. The face-lift is an excision of skin in the areas posterior to the temple, anterior to the pinna, and posterior to the pinna. Undermining of the sides of the face is done to pull the skin of the face upward to reduce the jowls that develop as a result of the aging process.

When it is necessary to remove tissues from the face because of deep malignancy the ability to select areas and levels of dissection for anatomical safety often is lost. The face-lift is a much safer procedure because the areas of incision as well as the levels of undermining can be selected carefully. Furthermore, the candidate can be chosen carefully.

THE LONG CONSULTATION

A minimum of one hour of the surgeon's time is required to cover the following: The patient should lose as much weight as is reasonably possible before the day of surgery. Forms of estrogen, including "the pill," and aspirin in any form should be omitted for two weeks preceding surgery. Patients taking an anticoagulant such as heparin or dicoumarol probably should not be candidates for the face-lift. The patient should shampoo and wash the face with Betadine shampoo for three days before the surgery.

With a proper face-lift, the patient will *not* look *many* years younger. The perfect face-lift makes the patient look as though he had a long, restful vacation. With time, the tissues again drift downward. The drifting is somewhat retarded by the diffuse scarring that develops beneath the undermining. In the patient with inherently good elastic fibers and collagen, the diminishing benefits are of value for five to eight years and proportionately less in the individual with sun-damaged collagen or hereditarily poor collagen and elastic fibers.

A clear, detailed surgical permit spelling out all possible complications should be signed and witnessed, together with a photographic release. Taking preoperative photographs, starkly realistic, is mandatory. General anesthesia cannot be given in the office setting without an anesthesiologist, and the patient must be informed of the effects of the analgesia that will be used. He must be told that the operation takes two to three hours. Shaving of the head is not necessary; hair clipping is described below.

The patient must be driven home and placed in a bed with a 30-degree elevation of the head. This is easily accomplished by folding blankets on or under

---

*Dr. Luikart is Assistant Clinical Professor of Medicine, Department of Dermatology, University of Southern California, Los Angeles.

the head of the mattress or using pillows. The patient must understand that the abrupt onset of pain means hemorrhage, which requires immediate surgical intervention. The telephone in the patient's area must be disconnected; the patient is to rest as much as is reasonably possible, with only bathroom privileges for 48 hours. A capable person must be in attendance to provide soft or liquid foods and to deter visitors. The patient can return to the office in 48 hours for removal of the pressure dressing. At that time, the nurse carefully combs out the hair with warm, soapy water and a wide-toothed comb. The face appears to be bruised and swollen. Usually the patient experiences temporary emotional depression. The patient may resume minimal activities.

The patient may gently comb the hair with warm water and a wide-toothed comb beginning the fourth day after surgery. The sutures anterior to the pinna will be removed in five to seven days. The patient can gently shampoo one week after surgery. The patient must be told that the ears may be numb and that a hair dryer must be warm, not hot. Makeup may be used after nine days. The stainless steel staples will be removed some ten to 15 days after the surgery.

ANALGESIA

A simple approach to analgesia is giving meperidine hydrochloride (Demerol) and Vistaril IM one-half hour before surgery. The dose is weight dependent, usually about 75 mg of Demerol and 25 mg of Vistaril. They have a synergistic benefit. The patient may also use Seconal orally one hour before coming to the office.

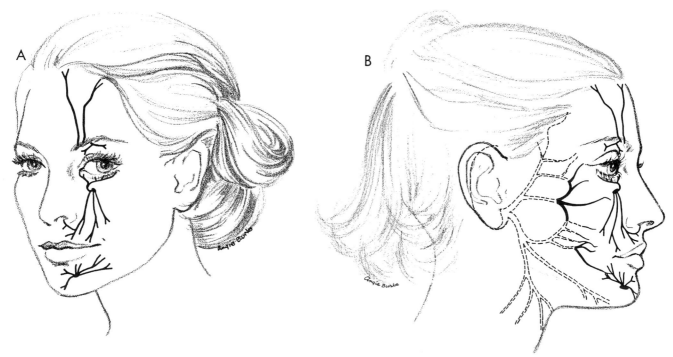

Fig 14–1.—**A,** schema of the emergence and distribution of the trigeminal nerve. **B,** schema of the emergence and distribution of the facial nerve. *Solid lines,* areas where the seventh nerve becomes more superficial. (From Luikart R.: The "Icononclast," a superb instrument for undermining. *J. Dermatol. Surg. Oncol.* 6:274–277, 1978. Used by permission.)

TABLE 14–1.—REVIEW OF SIGNIFICANT COMPLICATIONS REPORTED IN 3,595 FACE-LIFTS*

	CONWAY[1] (325 patients)	MCGREGOR[2] (524 patients)	BAKER[3] (1,500 patients)	LEIST[4] (324 patients)	THOMPSON[5] (922 patients)	AVERAGE
Hematoma (% patients)	6.6	8.1	15.6	5.9	5.0	10
Skin slough (% patients)	0.3	3.0	1.1	2.1	14.0	4.8
Nerve damage (% patients)	0.6	2.6	0.5	0.9	0.7	0.9

*From Luikart.[6] (Used by permission.)

ANATOMY

Figure 14–1 illustrates the distribution of the trigeminal and facial nerves that must be considered in any face-lift.

SEQUELAE

In five comprehensive articles constituting a study of 3,595 face-lifts,[1-5] the record shows an average incidence of 10% for hematomas, 4.8% for sloughs, and 0.9% for damage to the seventh motor nerve (Table 14–1).[6] These data indicate that blunt dissection when undermining is preferable to sharp dissection, since it reduces the hematoma problem while avoiding nerve damage. The blunt dissection should be extensive enough to produce the desired result without an excessively tight closure of the excisions.

When a nerve is severed, a neurosurgeon should be consulted to locate the ends and to perform a microanastomosis—within 48 hours if it is to be of value.

A hematoma discovered soon after closure can be drained with a #16 needle and controlled with pressure, or the flap must be opened for direct tie or electrocoagulation. Later, between the seventh and 14th days, the clots liquefy and can be drained through a large needle.

SURGICAL APPROACH

After a wide Betadine scrub of the incision areas, the nurse ties the hair into several strands, sprays the hair, tapes the margins, and positions the patient on the operating table with the head of the table elevated 20–30 degrees. The surgeon then plans his incisions, marks them with methylene blue or a similar material, and scissor trims away narrow zones of hair in those lines. Thorough local anesthesia of all areas involved in the procedure is induced by injecting 0.5% lidocaine with 1:200,000 solution of epinephrine. Waiting 20 minutes after this injection improves hemostasis a great deal, for small blood vessels are contracted. Full sterile technique is required. A frequently used incision is shown in Figure 14–2. This incision is in the natural crease anterior to the pinna and anterior to the tragus. It continues to the flat surface below the crease of the earlobe. On the posterior surface of the pinna, the incision starts in the crease and progresses onto the cartilage about 5 mm from the crease, as shown in the inset of Figure 14–2. This incision gradually curves posteriorly at the level of the external auditory meatus, crossing over the mastoid process.

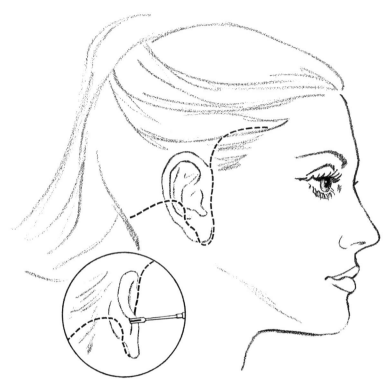

Fig 14–2.—Line of incision most frequently used for full face-lift. (From Luikart R.: The "Iconoclast," a superb instrument for undermining. *J. Dermatol. Surg. Oncol.* 6:274–277, 1978. Used by permission.)

Then the incision is extended into the lower margin of the hair in the occiput, to take up the slack as needed in each patient's neck.

Management of the cut to be made superior to the ear, through the temporal area, and gradually anterior toward the lateral forehead should be handled without initial incision because of the temporal artery. In addition to the methylene blue line, one may choose to create another, 1 mm deep, with a scalpel. Cautiously the depth of the incision is increased anterior to the pinna in the zone of the tragus until visualizing the thick fascia, which, at that position, is a combination of the joining of parotid fascia with the superficial musculoaponeurotic system (SMAS) of Mitz and Peyronie.[7] The length of this incision is cautiously extended above and below the initial entry for about 1 cm. With any blunt instrument, force the skin and dermis medially on the surface of SMAS to widen the 2-cm gap. Place an Iconoclast[6] (Fig 14–3) or blunt-nosed Metzenbaum scissors on the shiny SMAS. With the Iconoclast, the instrument can be pushed forward with ease at least 5 cm. With the power of the grip, the Iconoclast can easily be opened, undermining that fourth of the cheek with one maneuver. Withdraw the Iconoclast and through the same opening at the SMAS level force it onto the surface of the anterior auriculotemporal fascia as high up as necessary to extend the cut above the pinna. Press with the thumb against the skin hard enough to stabilize the posterior blade of the Iconoclast and force the anterior blade open with a gripping action, causing the anterior blade to glide over that fascia well beneath the hair papillae and above the temporal artery. Now, using curved scissors at a right angle to the surface, insert the lower blade gently into the undermined cavity. Scissor-cut safely the scalp tissue, freeing the upper aspect of this temporofrontal flap. With re-

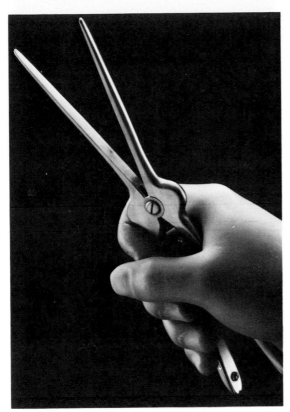

Fig 14–3.—The Iconoclast partly open. (From Luikart R.: The "Iconoclast," a superb instrument for undermining. *J. Dermatol. Surg. Oncol.* 6:274–277, 1978. Used by permission.)

peated insertion and opening of the Iconoclast, the undermining can be quickly finished to whatever extent is desired in the cheek. There always is an occasional fibrous strand between the dermis and SMAS that can be snipped free. Undermining inferior to the pinna, behind the pinna, over the mastoid process, and over the sternocleidomastoid muscle requires sharp dissection with a scalpel or scissors for a few centimeters. Then one can continue with the Iconoclast or Metzenbaum scissors down into the neck as indicated in Figure 14–4.

When advanced sagging warrants the risk, it is easy to continue the undermining toward or to the middle of the neck, to the nasolabial fold area, and approach the lateral eye and forehead areas. The most frequent injuries to the motor branches of the facial nerve occur to the temporofacial branch of this nerve, halfway between the superior aspect of the pinna and the lateral commissure of the eye, and to the marginal mandibular branch of this nerve along the margin of the ramus of the mandible.

Small bleeders at the margins of the incision are frequent. The majority of them stop bleeding in a few minutes without any intervention. Later, they can be electrocoagulated if necessary. Bleeders in the areas of sharp dissection may be numerous, and proper electrocoagulation or ties are mandatory. In the large flap areas undermined with scissors using the "spread-snip" technique, many bleeders occur. In the areas undermined with the Iconoclast, bleeders that demand attention are very few.

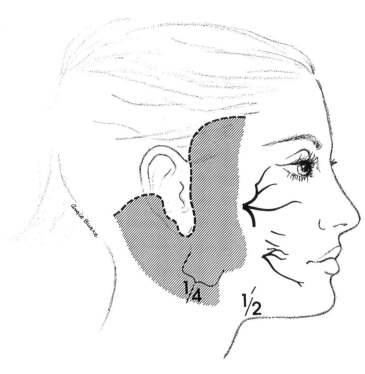

Fig 14–4.—*Shaded area* indicates the extent of moderate undermining. (From Luikart R.: The "Iconoclast," a superb instrument for undermining. *J. Dermatol. Surg. Oncol.* 6:274–277, 1978. Used by permission.)

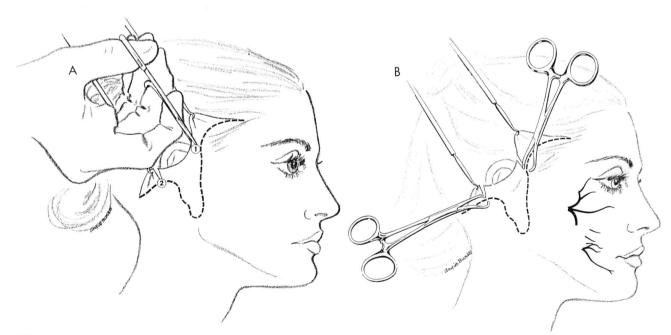

Fig 14–5.—**A,** determination of the positions of the first two key sutures. **B,** schema of temporary placement of key sutures with towel clips, which facilitates adjustment and readjustment as eventually needed. (From Luikart R.: The "Iconoclast," a superb instrument for undermining. *J. Dermatol. Surg. Oncol.* 6:274–277, 1978. Used by permission.)

Sharp dissection increases the possibilities of severing a nerve. It increases the number of severed blood vessels, which in turn increases the number of electrocoagulations, which itself also increases the possibility of accidental nerve damage. Finally, electrocoagulated vessels occasionally hemorrhage later.

After a dry field is obtained, the large flaps are moved with skin hooks. This maneuver enables the surgeon to visualize the most advantageous position for the flaps (Fig 14–5, A). The cuts are made to place the two key sutures (1 and 2 in Figure 14–5,A). These sutures then may be placed or the flaps may be held in position with towel clips (Fig 14–5,B). The overlaps of the flaps are scissored free as indicated in Figure 14–5,A.

At this point it is worthwhile to perform the same surgery on the other side of the face. This permits time for latent bleeders to make themselves apparent on the first side. Again, leaving the second side with key sutures or towel clips in place permits latent bleeders to become apparent on the second side while completing closure on the first side.

The large flap should fall into place anterior to the pinna with no pull. Exerting too much pull for closure above the pinna is an easy and common mistake, leading to temporary alopecia and widening of the scar line in the temporofrontal area. An extremely tight closure can produce ischemia and slough. The same problem exists in the occipital area, but the consequences of closing with too much tension are neither as frequent nor as visible.

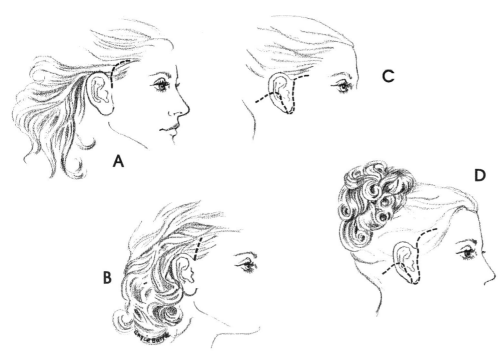

Fig 14–6.—A, line of incision for a moderate elevation of the cheek. **B,** line of a vertical incision to obtain pull in the forehead-eye area. **C,** line of incision for correction of sagging jowls, which is effective, but the scar will be exposed. **D,** recommended line of incision that is limited but well hidden, yet will give good improvement of cheek and jowl. (From Luikart R.: The ''Iconoclast,'' a superb instrument for undermining. *J. Dermatol. Surg. Oncol.* 6:274–277, 1978. Used by permission.)

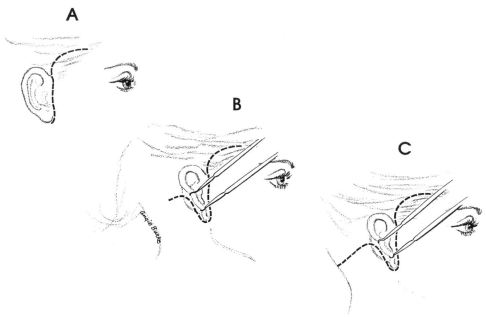

Fig 14–7.—**A,** a useful line of incision when no correction of the neck is needed. **B,** a limited incision posterior to the ear that is useful when correction of a neck is a minor problem. **C,** posterior extension of incision over and beyond the mastoid process preparatory to correction of a severe sagging in the neck. (From Luikart R.: The "Iconoclast," a superb instrument for undermining. *J. Dermatol. Surg. Oncol.* 6:274–277, 1978. Used by permission.)

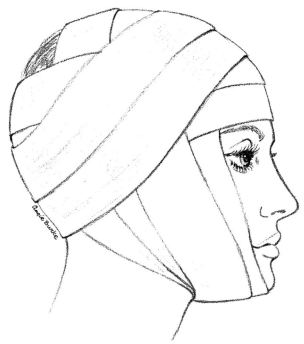

Fig 14–8.—The recommended postoperative pressure dressing. From Luikart R.: The "Iconoclast," a superb instrument for undermining. *J. Dermatol. Surg. Oncol.* 6:274–277, 1978. Used by permission.)

Closure anterior to the pinna can be done with a continuous subcutaneous 4-0 suture with only two or three interrupted 6-0 sutures. Closure behind the ear and over the mastoid process can be accomplished with interrupted 4-0 sutures with a couple of 3-0 sutures at the mastoid key pull area. The rest of the scalp areas can be quickly closed with stainless steel staples.

Figures 14–6 and 14–7 show some useful modifications of the face-lift in younger patients.

A good, firm dressing begins with soft cotton padding behind the pinna, Betadine solution and Polysporin ointment in small quantities on the lines of incision, tiny strips of Adaptic or Telfa over these lines of incision, followed by a good, firm wrapping with Ace bandages or Coban elastic bandage or tape (Fig 14–8). Some surgeons incorporate drains.

The stainless steel staples have been left in the scalp for more than three weeks without any apparent reaction or problem. The interrupted cutaneous sutures can be removed in seven to ten days.

REFERENCES

1. Conway H.: The surgical face lift: Rhytidectomy. *Plast. Reconstr. Surg.* 45:124–130, 1970.
2. McGregor M.W., Greenberg R.L.: *Rhytidectomy in the Unfavorable Result in Plastic Surgery: Avoidance and Treatment*. Boston, Little, Brown & Co., 1972, pp. 335–344.
3. Baker T.V., Gordon H.L., Mosienko P.: Rhytidectomy: A statistical analysis. *Plast. Reconstr. Surg.* 59:24–30, 1977.
4. Leist F.D., Masson J.K., Erick J.B.: A review of 324 rhytidectomies, emphasizing complications and patient dissatisfaction. *Plast. Reconstr. Surg.* 59:525–529, 1977.
5. Thompson D.P., Ashley F.L.: Face lift complications. *Plast. Reconstr. Surg.* 61:40–49, 1978.
6. Luikart R. II: The "Iconoclast," a superb instrument for undermining. *J. Dermatol. Surg. Oncol.* 6:274–277, 1978.
7. Mitz V., Peyronie M.: The superficial musculoaponeurotic system (SMAS) in the parotid and cheek area. *Plast. Reconstr. Surg.* 58:80–88, 1976.

15 / Treatment of Telangiectasias of the Legs

THE BEST SINGLE treatment of telangiectasias, or sunburst vessels, of the legs is sclerotherapy. It has been used for decades.[1-3] However, the emphasis on cosmesis in recent times has increased interest in this therapy. The use of the hyfrecator and epilating needle, which is so successful on the face, chest, and arms, does not produce the desired results for the sunburst vessels on the legs. Often, there are white punctate scars and some of the vessels shrink down with a linear atrophic scar. When effective, the laser beam produces multiple, round, white, unnatural-looking, and, we think, unattractive marks.

SCLEROSING SOLUTION

The classic sclerosing mixture has been a 16%–24% sodium chloride solution, with 20% being most commonly used. (Sodium chloride concentrate, 23.4% is available from McGaw, Cutter, Abbott, and Ivenex laboratories in rubber-stoppered vials from 30 to 100 ml.) Sometimes the addition of heparin, 100 units/ml of sodium chloride solution, helps prevent intravascular clotting, which may lead to a temporary blue-black linear appearance. The heparin does not alter the rate of success.

A variety of hyperosmolar solutions formerly was available commercially. These were made up with salts and sugars. The increased hyperosmolarity from the addition of the sugar was beneficial, while the amount of actual sodium chloride injected was reduced. This was believed to reduce the chance of skin slough.

Another technique was to use Sotradecol foam. The regular Sotradecol designed for varicose veins was shaken to produce a foamy top. The top was aspirated into a 1-ml tuberculin-type syringe and injected into the telangiectasias by the same technique as with the other methods discussed below. Because Sotradecol is so irritating to the vessel walls, the foam was a clever method of exposing the vessel endothelium to small amounts of the material. A recent report suggests that injecting only 0.1 ml of Sotradecol liquid per site gives excellent results.[3] The solution should be diluted 4 to 1. A more modern sclerosing agent is aethoxysclerol (hydroxypolyethoxy-dodecane), which is not available in the United States, but has been used widely throughout Europe. For use in sunburst telangiectasias, it is diluted with normal saline solution to a concentration of 0.25% or used in 0.5% or 1.0% concentration for resistant vessels. However, it may be necessary to treat again in 2 to 4 weeks.

Careful and reported scientific comparisons among these various agents are not known to us. We must rely on clinical impressions from the physicians who have been using these agents for many years; physicians whom we be-

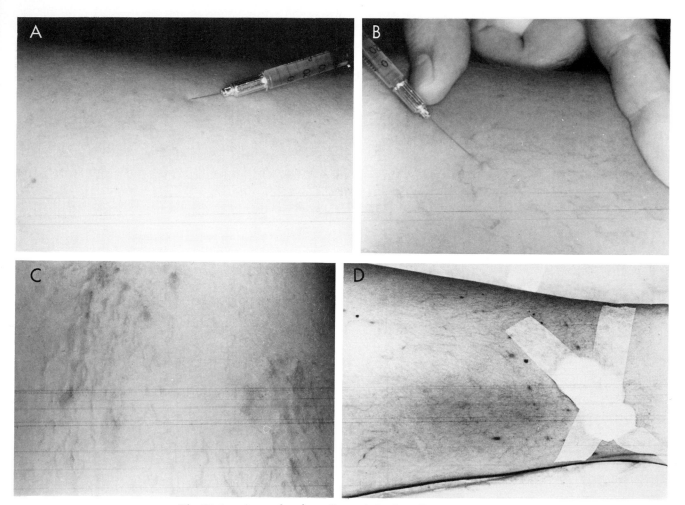

Fig 15–1.—A, angle of needle on injection. **B,** preinjection.
C, immediately after injection, showing swelling of vessels. **D,** pressure pad applied to prevent back-bleeding.

lieve are careful in their work, observations, and reporting. As best as we can tell from limited information, concentrated sodium chloride, sodium chloride plus various sugars, or aethoxysclerol all appear to have about the same degree of effectiveness and side effects.

TECHNIQUE

The instrumentation and technique of injection vary slightly among physicians. The standard method is to draw the sclerosing solution into a 1-ml tuberculin-type syringe with a 1/2-in., 30-gauge, disposable needle. The needle is bent to approximately a 45-degree angle with the bevel of the needle facing upward (Fig 15–1,A). The needle then is placed flat on the skin surface with its tip approximately 4.0–5.0 mm from the chosen vessel. Pressure is applied forward rather than downward. This causes the tip of the needle to slip slowly into the skin and into the vessel, which is part of the subepidermal plexus. An extremely small amount of the solution is injected into the vessel. The physician watches closely so that the slightest bit of blanching as the clear sclerosing solution displaces the blood is observed (Fig 15–1,B). If the vessel is well cannulated, the solution is gently pushed through the vessel; many vessels in the surrounding area may blanch. With experience, the key vessel of a large arbor of vessels often can be distinguished. If this trunk vessel is cannulated and injected, an entire sunburst may blanch. The material is injected through the vessel as long as it remains patent. After 0.1–0.5 ml of sclerosing solution has passed the vessels, they become irritated and hyperemic (Fig 15–1,C). This is the natural end point and the desired one for all injections. However, often the vessel wall will rupture, or the unsteadiness of the physician may move the needle out of the vessel.

The danger of infiltrating the solutions into the surrounding tissues is variable. Occasionally, a hyperpigmented macule will develop at this infiltrated spot. It is our experience that such macules usually fade within six months. There are some vessels that are trunk vessels that leak the solution as we are injecting. Nevertheless, we continue to inject because the rest of the arbor is blanching. A small amount of infiltrated substance does not seem to leave any residual damage, and the treatment of the entire sunburst is well worth the trade-off. Extravasation of larger amounts can produce small white scars. Rarely, in the pretibial area significant scars have been seen. Injecting with plain lidocaine to dilute the amount of solution extravasated often is helpful.

The patient experiences only slight pain during standard injection. No one ever has asked that we stop and no one ever has seemed to be in any great discomfort. The injection sessions can be designed according to a period of time (5 minutes, 30 minutes, 45 minutes) or quadrants (lower leg, upper leg, etc.). The division will be determined by how the physician wants to charge for the procedure and by how many vessels are to be treated on any given patient. We generally start with the vessels on the lower legs and then work superiorly.

With experience, it is possible to deposit a tiny amount of the solution just exterior to the extremely tiny blood vessels. This should not be attempted until one is comfortable with the standard procedure.

Another technique is to use a 1-in., 30-gauge needle on a 3-ml disposable syringe. Because of its length and flexibility, the physician can twist, arc, and curve the tip of the needle into vessels at various directions and angles to the skin. Other physicians prefer the tiny 32- or 33-gauge, 1/4-in. needles. The 32-gauge needles currently are available from surgical supply sources (Alpro Supply Company, Farmingdale, NY; Robbins Instrument Company, Chatham, NJ; and George Tieman & Company, Long Island City, NY.) They also can be made specially by major needle manufacturers.

Once a "feel" for the technique has been achieved, your success rate can be increased further by switching to the following technique. Using the 1/2-in., 30-gauge or the 1/4-in., 32- or 33-gauge needle bent to the proper angle, insert the whole bevel of the needle into the skin approximately 5.0 mm from the vessel you wish to enter. With thumb or index finger, apply the slightest amount of pressure to the plunger. The pressure should be so light that the normal tissue turgor allows no fluid to enter the skin. Maintain pressure and advance the needle as described above. As soon as the bevel enters the vessel, the low intraluminal pressure and flow of blood compared to the static turgor of the tissue around the vessel will allow instant movement of sclerosant into the vessel, clearing out the blood. The appropriate amount of material then may be injected. This takes practice but will increase your rate of success. At no time should sclerosant material be injected into the tissue.

Still another variation is to use a 3.0-ml syringe with 2 1/2 ml of solution and 0.5 cc of air. The injections always are made with the needle pointing upward. The air enters first, and if the vessels blanch owing to the air in the vessels pushing away the blood, the sclerosant is injected. If the vessels do not blanch and air is injected intradermally, the needle is withdrawn and a new vessel is selected for injection. This technique is favored by its users as a method to prevent sclerosant from being injected outside the vessels. The technique has been used successfully for years without evidence of air embolism. The users generally limit the amount of air injected per session to approximately 5 cc. Past forensic pathologic studies have suggested that in excess of 250 cc of IV air is needed to produce death in human beings. We do not specifically recommend this method, since we have not used it, but it has been recommended by practitioners we trust. Which method each practitioner selects is an individual decision based on potential benefits, risks, and experience.

After injecting the vessels, immediately apply pressure with a cotton ball or

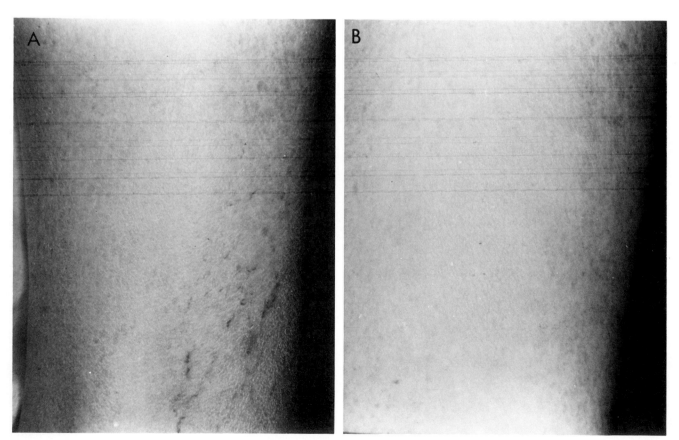

Fig 15–2.—A, before injection. **B,** after treatment complete.

gauze at that site (Fig 15–1,D). An assistant can do this. A small cotton ball with a piece of tape firmly over it will hold pressure over the vessel, help prevent the vessel from filling with blood (which will dilute the irritant effect of the sclerosant), and help prevent leakage of blood into the dermis. At the end of the session, it is wise to wrap the legs with some sort of elastic gauze, such as Coban. The dressing is placed right over the cotton balls so that point pressure is maintained over the injection sites. This helps prevent postinjection bleeding and should help the overall rate of success, since it prevents the vessels from filling again. Ambulation is allowed on the first day, although vigorous sports activity is not recommended for several days. The dressings are removed in one to two days, and the patients should be advised that there will be varying degrees of ecchymotic discolorations to the legs. The vessels seem to fade in the first two to three weeks postinjection; some require up to three months before fading (Fig 15–2 and Plate IV, D and E). Vessels that remain patent can be reinjected at two-week intervals.

Regardless of which instrumentation and which technique the physician uses, it is a good idea to discuss with the patient the unpredictability of the results. We ask the patients to share in the risk by saying that the size of the vessels in their own telangiectasias has a lot to do with determining the success of the treatment. We point out that the success is based on the fact that their vessels will become irritated and will swell shut and then not later recanalize. It makes patients more likely to accept the fact that sometimes only 50%–75% of those vessels injected will close down successfully.

MECHANISM OF ACTION

There are four theories about the mechanism of action of the sclerosing solution. One theory was discussed above: the vessel endothelium is irritated and swells shut and does not recanalize because it is a low-pressure system. Another theory is that a clot will form and, with its resolution over several weeks, the vessels do not recanalize. A third theory is that the vessels do recanalize but, because of the inflammation of the endothelium, gradually close off, and there is an observable, progressive decrease in color as they gradually fade. The fourth theory is that paravascular damage results in microscopic fibrosis, which slowly closes the vessels. Whatever the mechanism of action, we believe this to be a successful and safe treatment. Whether new vessels recur or whether old vessels open also is supposition. We tell our patients that they will need a "touch-up" one to five years later. Some women come in each spring before the bathing suit season to have us treat new or recurring vessels because some vessels take up to three months to resolve.

SIDE EFFECTS

The side effects include small, white, depressed scars from extravasation of the material. This is rare but has happened occasionally. We know of one case of significant pretibial scarring. More commonly, spots of hyperpigmentation at the sites of injection appear, but are almost always temporary (Fig 15–3). We have not performed biopsies on these to see whether they are hemosiderin, increased melanin in the epidermis, or melanin in the upper dermis.

Occasionally, an injected vessel will form a black linear clot. This may cause

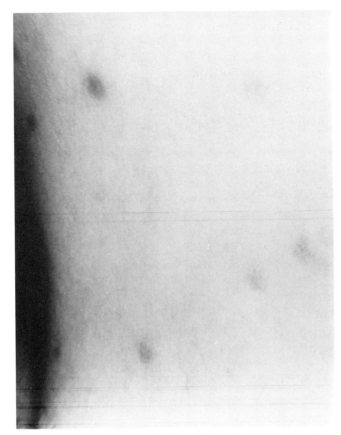

Fig 15–3.—Brown spots postinjection. They should slowly disappear.

continuous, low-grade pain. Treatment is to nick the skin and vessel very superficially with a #11 blade and express the linear clot with cotton-tipped applicators. Relief of pain is instantaneous. Finger pressure supplies hemostasis if any is needed.

Theoretically, there would be a problem with injection of the concentrated solution of sodium chloride into patients who have hypertension or severe cardiovascular disease. However, if the total dose of 20% sodium chloride solution does not exceed 5–10 ml given over a 20- to 30-minute period, we are told by cardiologists that there is little chance of complication. However, patients with severe cardiovascular disease or severe hypertension usually are not seeking treatment for the fine vessels in the legs.

SUMMARY

This is an extremely tedious and time-consuming procedure. We try to have these patients scheduled for early in the morning so that our hands and our patients are the steadiest. The real reward from this procedure is the salutary effect on the appearance of the legs. The patients almost always are gratified. There seems to be a minimum of serious risk, and the side effects are transitory.

REFERENCES

1. Foley W.T.: The eradication of venous blemishes. *Cutis* 15:665–668, 1975.
2. Weissberg D.: Treatment of varicose veins by compression sclerotherapy. *Surg. Gynecol. Obstet.* 151:353–356, 1980.
3. Shields J.L., Jansen T.G.: Therapy for superficial telangiectasias of the lower extremities. *J. Dermatol. Surg. Oncol.* 8:857–860, 1982.

16 / Corrective Makeup Techniques: A Case Study Approach

SUSAN CRISTIAN*

THERE ARE FEW PEOPLE who, after a car accident, would suggest that the collision shop merely remove the dents, fill in the cracks, smooth the rough edges, and return the vehicle. Although the more difficult part of reconstruction and correction is finished, the work is not complete. Only after the paint is dried and the glaze hardened will the car appear unblemished. Beneath the paint, the scars and results of repair are hidden. From the outside, the illusion is one of newness. The work of a physician and corrective cosmetic consultant is similar. Makeup is a natural extension of the corrective process.

The assumption that cosmetics are an appropriate adjunct to facial surgery is not without basis. Research paradigms examining the effects of physical attractiveness have manipulated appearance through the use of makeup. These studies demonstrate that facial appearance is a significant variable in evaluations of interpersonal attraction, others' perceptions of physical attractiveness, and self-perception.[1] More recent evidence suggests that use of cosmetics leads to more favorable appearance and personality ratings by others.[2] Makeup makes a difference. Together, the combined strategy of surgery and cosmetics minimizes the effects of aging on the skin. The result is a happier, more attractive patient.

This chapter examines the nature and scope of work performed by a corrective consultant through a content analysis of procedures used in four different cases. The extent to which these services overlap the medical field and are available to physicians also is discussed.

OVERVIEW

Clients who secure the services of a corrective cosmetic consultant can do so in several ways. Ideally, a well-trained consultant can work in a physician's office. Although the consultant can work in conjunction with several areas of medical specialization, dermatology offers the greatest opportunity to integrate science with artistry and extensive knowledge of an annual $5–10-billion cosmetics industry. Areas that have been identified as helpful to the physician include providing patients with routine, time-consuming instruction on skin care and treatment procedures. Through knowledge of cosmetic ingredients, skin irritants can be identified more easily and replaced by compatible products. Therapeutic makeup and techniques of application for nonsurgical prob-

*Corrective Cosmetic Consultant, Campus Commons Medical Plaza, Sacramento, California.

lems, such as birthmarks and pigmentation, can be provided also.[3] Working together, more answers are available to the greater number of questions that patients ask. Independent consultants work in their own offices within a medical complex. Most clients are obtained through referrals from dermatologists, plastic surgeons, and otolaryngologists.

When a client first visits a corrective cosmetic consultant, the patient must voice his concerns about his appearance. Sometimes an individual will be the victim of overexpectation, dissatisfied with the slowness of healing after cosmetic or reconstructive surgery. Postoperative makeup techniques enable these patients to cope with normal skin discolorations and edema during the healing period. This encouragement often allays doubts about the success of surgery, and because facial appearance is improved, patients tend to worry less. Other clients express a lack of enthusiasm for cosmetics but perceive a need for coverage of a specific problem. Many are knowledgeable about common over-the-counter products but recognize a need for more occlusive makeup. For whatever reason—pigmentation, trauma, postsurgical discolorations, scarring, keloids, etc.—clients seek an improved appearance.

There are two basic approaches to successful cosmetic application. Coverage often is all that is needed to camouflage facial imperfections. Where structural defects and uneven skin texture are present, optical illusions draw attention away from blemished areas to more attractive features. Each client goes through three stages of cosmetic improvement. First, the skin is cleansed thoroughly and given sunscreen protection. Second, camouflage makeup is applied and covered with a foundation product. The occlusive cosmetics mute discolorations and are placed only on the marred area. The foundation base is applied over the entire facial region to eliminate lines of demarcation caused by the corrective product. The result is even, natural color. Finally, enhancement makeup adds color to the eye, nose, cheek, and lip regions and creates optical illusions where needed. The four cases described emphasize camouflage procedures.

Case 1—Trauma

The first case is that of an 18-year-old woman who suffered multiple windshield lacerations that required skin grafting. Instruction on corrective makeup was given four weeks postoperatively (Fig 16–1,A). The goal in this case was natural coverage that would allow the client to appear in public without feeling self-conscious.

Scars are covered in the following manner. After thorough cleansing and sunscreen protection, a yellow muting cream is applied in a thin line over the wounded area. A cotton swab is used to bring the cream to the edges of the affected region.

Following coverage, a foundation makeup is applied with a cosmetic sponge. A foundation base is a slightly pigmented cosmetic that is designed to cover minor flaws and uneven color in the skin. When applied properly, foundations provide a neutral background for later enhancement makeup.

In this case, the product used was Physician's Formula *L.E. Velvet Film.** This

---

*The particular foundation product that is recommended to a patient can vary greatly. Consideration is given to skin type, skin age, the presence of wrinkles, and any prior facial elective surgery. Esthetics and financial ability also are important. Mention of a product, therefore, is not a general endorsement for all patients.

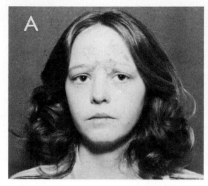 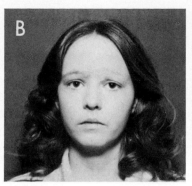 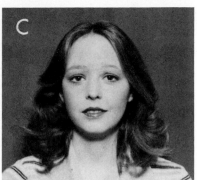

Fig 16–1.—Corrective makeup of a patient who suffered multiple facial lacerations. **A,** appearance before makeup. **B,** appearance following use of a makeup sponge to apply foundation. **C,** cosmetics and color added to foundation.

foundation is a water-based cream cosmetic that offers good coverage and wide availability at a reasonable price. Physical and chemical sunscreens in this product give added protection to wearers (sun protective factor [SPF] = 15). Titanium dioxide, the active ingredient that gives the product its "covering power" is more effective than zinc oxide, which often is used in other foundations for the same purpose.[4] A cake makeup such as this is good in trauma cases because it it easy both to apply and to remove. Skin that is recovering from the shock of injury often is quite tender. More important than a particular product, however, is the method of application.

Proper technique is important so that the corrective underlayer will not be disturbed. The general rule is that no makeup ever should be rubbed into the skin. By using a cosmetic sponge, foundation can be applied to be both flattering and effective. The sponge used is a soft, white, polyfoam applicator, unlike the natural-looking cleansing sponges that have visible holes. After putting makeup on a clean sponge, rest the sponge on the skin and gently roll it from left to right and back again using light pressure. The sponge then is repositioned and the method repeated until the entire facial area is covered. When this is completed, the face is ready for enhancement makeup (Fig 16–1,B). Later, cosmetics add color and give the client a natural, youthful appearance (Fig 16–1,C).

For male clients who have little natural inclination toward makeup, a foundation base usually is eliminated. Unless the marred area is extensive, a small amount of muting cream is placed over the scar and proves sufficient. Using a cotton swab, the cream is smudged slightly around the edges to blend with the skin. In this instance, the entire procedure (cleansing, sunscreen protection, and coverage) takes only minutes, and male clients seem willing to trade a little time for this improved appearance.

Case 2—Vitiligo

Recommendations for cosmetic correction in vitiligo cases vary according to the intensity of the discoloration. The 45-year-old woman in this case suffered minor facial hypopigmentation (Plate IV,F). In this instance, use of Physician's Formula *L.E. Velvet Film* proved to be effective. Application with a sponge allowed for good coverage and control of the amount of makeup applied (Plate IV,G).

Often in hyperpigmentation and hypopigmentation cases it is difficult to find a cosmetic that closely resembles the skin's natural color. When this occurs, one should choose a color that is one shade darker than areas in which melanin production is normal. This allows for the blending of makeup along lines of demarcation and a slightly heavier cosmetic application in troublesome areas. If the color of the foundation is too light, a pasty, masked appearance is created.

A second difficulty arises when vitiliginous skin extends to the neck region. It is not recommended to apply cosmetics beyond the chin line because makeup will collect in neck creases. This not only mitigates cosmetic improvement but can cause stains to clothing that are difficult to remove. The best solution is to suggest that clients wear clothing that covers the neck area. When this is not feasible, makeup should be applied only around the borders of the skin lesions, where it can be blended. The goal here is not to cover the skin but to lessen lines of demarcation.

Where skin lesions are completely depigmented, it is necessary to use a more occlusive makeup followed by a foundation base. Lydia O'Leary *Covermark* provides excellent coverage and can appear natural if applied properly. Another advantage of this product is its staying power: once applied, it will last throughout the day. Application technique is important because improper use can lead to a heavy, artificial appearance. Clients suffering from vitiligo, severe body scarring, and port-wine birth marks are advised to strive for 80% coverage in use of this product. When this is done, secondary enhancement makeup will achieve its most flattering effectiveness. The two different types of cosmetics will complement each other rather than compete visually for the attention of the viewer.

Another way to improve the appearance of vitiligo is through complete avoidance of the sun or use of broad-spectrum sunscreens. This will cause normal pigmentation to fade in light-skinned persons, making the contrast between affected and unaffected areas less noticeable. Sunscreen protection also is important as a means of protecting lesions from sunburn.

Products that stain the skin are another option. The active ingredient DHA (dihydroxyacetone) stains the skin a yellowish brown. Although it may accomplish this purpose, it is difficult to achieve a satisfactory cosmetic effect. Rather than dye the whole skin to look like a tan, in vitiligo cases the goal is to dye areas that lack pigmentation so that they match normal skin. The process is tedious; "color fades after two days and is lost completely after eight to 14 days as the superficial cells of the skin naturally rub off."[5] DHA also provides no sunscreen protection and sunburn can occur. Other dyes can be helpful with specific patients.

Case 3—Postsurgical Discoloration

Discolorations secondary to surgery can be easily camouflaged. The bruises on this 58-year-old woman (Fig 16–2,A) are the result of a full face-lift and blepharoplasty.

In this case (see Fig 16–2,A), yellow muting cream was applied to discolorations seven days postoperatively. A sponge is used on large areas but a cotton swab works best around the eye region. To prepare the face for enhancement

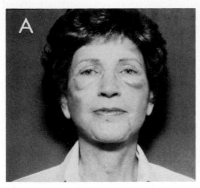 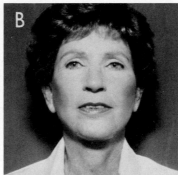

Fig 16–2.—Camouflage of postsurgical discoloration. **A,** bruises resulting from full face-lift and blepharoplasty in a 58-year-old woman. **B,** appearance seven days postoperatively, after application of a yellow muting cream and enhanced makeup.

makeup *Countess Isserlyn Creme* by Alexandra de Markoff is applied with a sponge. This product works well on more mature skins; its high moisture content allows for good spreadability and ease of application.

Because puffy, swollen eyes are common at this time, the corrective process includes enhancement makeup that will shift emphasis away from the eyelid to the eye itself. The basic rule of optical illusion comes into play: light brings features forward and dark causes features to recede. Thus, a dark, matte shadow functions to diminish the swollen appearance (Fig 16–2,B).[6]

After the eye and face have regained a normal appearance, changes in makeup often are necessary. Reshaping of eyebrows and cosmetic adjustments for asymmetric eyelid creases sometimes are necessary. A more youthful appearance also is greatly enhanced by more youthful makeup. Patients who anticipate these changes tend to accept a more active role in their appearance and are less likely to assign to the surgeon responsibility for minor cosmetically correctable flaws.

Case 4—Chemical Peel

Clients who have undergone chemical peels or dermabrasion seem to experience the most postoperative discomfort and emotion. For them, the procedures can be painful and traumatic. Healing is slow, and on certain days they believe that their skin is worse, not better. The importance of makeup at this time cannot be underestimated. If it is recognized that minimal use is best during the healing phase, cosmetics can improve appearance and can extend a patient's patience. Clients who wear makeup seem to exhibit less anxiety. They are able to do other things besides waiting for nature to complete the healing process.

Makeup may be applied as early as seven days postoperatively when necessary, but it is better to wait 12 days. These clients routinely are advised to use sunscreen protection in a nonalcohol base because the skin of chemical peel and dermabrasion clients is so sensitive at this time.

The woman in this case is shown 14 days after a chemical peel (Plate IV,H). Use of sunscreen protection and a muting cream protects the skin and eliminates redness. Alexandra de Markoff *Countess Isserlyn Creme* then is applied, using the same techniques described previously. Lines of demarcation are eliminated, and a natural appearance is created (Plate IV,I).

The four cases described are brief examples of the work performed by a corrective cosmetic consultant. Although there is a great need for these services throughout the country, there is no formal training program that gives consultants the extensive background needed for this work.

It is true that a large amount of glamour is associated with the skin care industry, but glamour assumes the option of "normalcy" should the wearer decide not to be cloaked in the lotions, creams, and colors of cosmetics. Clients who come to my office do not always have that option. They seek a normal appearance, and the little magic that helps bring this about can be achieved only through corrective cosmetics.

REFERENCES

1. Graham J.A., Jouhar A.J.: Cosmetics considered in the context of physical attractiveness: A review. *Int. J. Cosmet. Sci.* 2:77–101, 1980.
2. Graham J.A., Jouhar A.J.: The effects of cosmetics on person perception. *Int. J. Cosmet. Sci.* In press.
3. Pugliese P.T.: A physician's view of the emerging skin care market. *Cosmet. Toil.* 94: 26–7, 1979.
4. Conry T.: *Consumer's Guide to Cosmetics.* New York, Anchor Books, 1980, p. 215.
5. Hulme J.R.: Suntan, sunburn and sunscreen applications. *Nurs. Times* 71: 1200–1201, 1975.
6. Cristian S.F.: Corrective eyelid makeup techniques for cosmetic surgery, in Putterman A.M. (ed.): *Cosmetic Oculoplastic Surgery.* New York, Grune & Stratton. In press.

17 / Cosmetics

THE USE OF cosmetics seems to be programmed into our genetic nature. Human beings first want to look normal, i.e., like members of their peer group. They then want to look better than their peers and add beauty or glamour as defined by their cultural environment. In the cosmetics world, we call the first process normalization and the second process enhancement.

COSMETIC TERMS

"Normalization" means to transform variations in human color or form, through the use of external applications, to the norm. The typical example would be eliminating a pink-purple nevus flammeus on the face.

Enhancement is to take a normal appearance and add color or the appearance of form. Enhancement also can be a second step in normalization, in which the person with the nevus flammeus covers the objectionable color, then enhances the rest of the appearance with appropriate cosmetic techniques. Enhancement includes all of the coloring agents for eyelids, face, and body, as well as the variety of prosthetic devices that may be attached, such as eyelashes and fingernails. Frequently, the same types of products are used for both normalization and enhancement, the difference being in the amount and type of color in the product.

NORMAL APPLICATION STEPS

The typical cosmetic application as commonly done by girls and women consists of six or seven basic steps. Step 1 is to remove old makeup, dirt, sebum, and loose stratum corneum cells. The skin is cleansed usually with soap and water. For women whose skin does not tolerate even mild cleansers, such as Dove, Neutrogena, or Dermage Washable Cleanser, creams or lotions are used. The oil phase of the cream or lotion acts as a solvent for sebum and cosmetic oils, and the emulsion in creams and lotions allows sebum to be emulsified and carried away with dirt and loosened cells of the stratum corneum. The cream or lotion can be wiped off with tissue or simply rinsed with water. The method an individual uses depends on the inherent dryness or oiliness of the skin; there is no single best method.

Step 2 is to use a toner or freshener. Basically, these are solvents that have additional cleansing action. They are also used to remove excess oil from step 1, since tissue wiping and rinsing with water will not remove excess oil. The person using step 2 learns to balance the amount of cream used in step 1 against the amount of freshener-toner used in step 2. Toners generally include a substance with a high evaporative rate to give a sensation of cooling or immediate change in the skin, analogous to the "fresh" feeling after application of aftershave lotion. The use of cream in step 1 and toner in step 2 gives a feel to the skin that the person will enjoy.

Step 3 is application of a cream or lotion moisturizer.

Step 4 is application of a foundation in the form of a cream or lotion. These products are colored, powdered pigments mixed with an emulsion to make the pigment adhere to the skin surface. Another eight or ten chemicals are needed to obtain the desired qualities, such as even application, proper feel on fingers, proper feel on the face, even dispersion of pigment through the product, etc. Although foundations comprise powdered pigment, water, and oil, they are true masterpieces of the cosmetic chemist's art.

Foundation is applied by the fingers or cosmetic sponge according to dictates of the cyclical nature of fashion in cosmetics. The only truly proper method is that which gives the desired look and feel. Finger application most often is used; use of cosmetic sponges makes for a thicker application and frequently more even application for certain situations, particularly those in which normalization is being accomplished. Cosmetic sponges were criticized some years ago because of bacterial and mold growth in the pores of the sponge. They seem to be making a comeback. In makeup for movies, stage, or television, professional makeup artists use a fine-grade (pore) cosmetic sponge to obtain the most even application and the specific desired thickness for the effect desired.

Step 5 is the application of blusher to the cheeks to simulate the rosy cheek appearance or a nonanatomical application to obtain a specific effect, such as to draw attention upward, to widen the appearance of the upper face, to camouflage acne scars, etc. Blushers are pink-red cosmetics and come in cream, lotion, brush-on powder, and stick forms. Some blushers are meant to be applied with a sweeping motion. Many women who do not use foundation apply blusher in this manner to give the pink look to the malar area. When using cream blusher, a more sophisticated approach is to apply blusher with the fingertips in a dotting-patting motion. This allows the blusher to be more easily blended in and actually become a part of the foundation. For women who are particularly fastidious about the intensity of blusher or who like to have more blusher anteriorly with a trailing off of color toward the lateral malar area, finger application provides this result. Powder blushers also give excellent application control.

Step 6 is the application of powder to set the foundation. Essentially, the powder converts the cream or lotion foundation to an elegant paste, which insures better retention of foundation and, therefore, better color quality on the skin. One only has to think of products such as zinc oxide to appreciate that pastes adhere well to the skin. The paste we are describing is, of course, a most refined preparation, but the pharmaceutical principles are the same. The powder can be applied with cotton balls, which is the most hygienic method. Women should put an excessive amount of powder on the cotton balls, since they do not carry a large amount of powder to the skin. Far more effective is the use of a powder puff, which is patted on the skin and places more powder over the foundation. Powder puffs periodically fall into disuse because of the possibility of bacteria and fungus growth in and on the puff owing to accumulation of lotion or cream. Professional makeup artists working in stage, screen, and television use puffs. Complaints that makeup does not last long enough are usually attributable to insufficient powder being applied to set the foundation.

Powders come in many varieties. The tan tones desired are obtained by the foundation color. The powder is sheer, essentially maintaining the same tone as that gained by application of the foundation. Powders, however, also can be tinted, since the tint materials in most makeups are colored powders. Tans, pinks, reds, etc., can be added to a powder to produce a highlighting shade that is additive to the foundation color.

Step 7 is used by women with fine wrinkles. The application of the powder tends to accent wrinkles. A small amount of moisturizer is applied with the fingertip to areas where wrinkles show. This step softens the effect of the powder so that wrinkles are less apparent, yet the makeup lasts and looks natural.

At the end of the day, makeup is removed using soap and water, Dermage Washable Cleanser, lotions, or creams. Makeup that has been applied for normalization generally must be removed by some type of cream. Again, the analogy to zinc oxide paste (ointment) is that water is not very effective in removing a paste. Therefore, oil must be added in the form of a cream to overcome the paste effect and produce a mixture that can be removed with tissue and further cleansed with soap and water, a washable cleanser, or freshener (toner) to solubilize the oil. The best procedure for each patient depends on the type of foundation and the amount of powder applied. The most effective makeup remover is to apply a heavy cream and remove it with tissue. Then remove remaining makeup with soap and water or with toner. In addition to makeup removal, this generally leaves the skin with a smooth, fresh feel.

SELECTION OF COSMETICS

Selection of a makeup line depends on your individual practice and the particular women whom you advise. Because one of us (T.A.T.) was involved in the development of a new makeup line as elegant as other makeups but having specific medical qualities, he, of course, favors Dermage cosmetics. The advantages of Dermage cosmetics are three. First, all products are tested to have the lowest irritability possible. Several other cosmetic lines do cause low-grade irritation, particularly in postoperative skin. Although Dermage itself could irritate some skin it has the lowest potential to do so. Second, all products are tested for comedogenicity; that is, no product is released unless it can be shown in both laboratory and human tests not to produce plugging of the pores and blackheads. Third, the formulations remain stable. It is common for cosmetic companies to change their products as frequently as every six to 12 months while the names stay the same. However, the cosmetic that was recommended last year now actually may be significantly different. Dermage maintains the same cosmetics, or, if any change must be made, various tests prove that the lowest possible irritability and noncomedogenicity are repeated.

Recently, Dermage has introduced a new cream sunscreen foundation that is ideal for routine use and for the post operative period. It has a SPF of 20–26 and has a moisturizing capability equal to other products which are labeled only as moisturizer creams. This product has the usual Dermage properties of hypoallergenicity, hypoirritability, and no comedogenicity, but also has the special feature of having its moisturizing effect last for several days.

Usually, available modern cosmetics normalize almost all problems, provided that a cosmetic sponge is used and attention to details observed. For occasional patients, a thicker preparation made by Lydia O'Leary is excellent. This contains greater amounts of particulate material, which will provide greater coverage. The trade-off is better coverage for more of a "made-up" look. The patient with a skin defect needs to decide whether the end result should be the greatest amount of coverage, using Lydia O'Leary makeup, or compromise for a more "light makeup" look.

OTHER COSMETIC PRODUCTS

Lipsticks essentially are a combination of pigments, oils, waxes, and other ingredients to make up the lipstick base. In the past stains were added to give lipstick the lasting quality that women appreciate throughout the day. The stains, however, were coal tar derivatives and a common cause of allergy in lipsticks, so they are eliminated in modern lipsticks. If the same color quality is obtained safely; however, the lipstick must be reapplied during the day. One trick in prolonging the effectiveness of lipstick and also to make it "kissproof" (i.e., it will not readily come off on contact) is to apply powder over the lipstick in the same manner that powder is applied over foundation base. Lipstick fashion changes so rapidly that it is impossible to recommend specific brands.

Eye makeup consists of eye shadow, mascara, liner, and pencil. It is most important for the physician to know that studies have shown that most of the benefits of a totally made-up face come from eye makeup. Your office person recommending makeup or your makeup consultant should be acutely aware of this fact. The studies were done with the end point being enhancement by makeup rather than normalization. Therefore, proper individualized use of eye makeup can maximize your surgical result. The most common causes of allergy in eye makeup are from mascara and eye shadow. Work is being done to try to provide a truly hypoallergenic mascara, and it is hoped that this will be available in the near future. Shades of color, shininess, iridescence, etc., are rapidly changing styles, and, again, specific brands are not recommended. However, the physician should realize that nearly all the major manufacturers produce hypoallergenic cosmetics. If a woman is using an off-brand or small-company cosmetics line and develops allergy or irritation, she can try several other lines with specific medical advantages or the major brands. If there is mascara allergy, the woman may find a nonirritating product suitable for her in any line.

COSMETIC "SYSTEMS"

Many "systems" are recommended by cosmetics companies. Each company states that it has its own special system and that only its system and complete line of products work together. Actually, the majority of American women seem to mix brands to obtain the individualized cosmetic effects that they desire. The claim by some manufacturers that only their products can be used and that they must not be mixed with others is not true in our experience. That claim sells more cosmetics for the particular company but does not really render the best service for each woman who needs individualized cosmetics.

MODERN TRENDS

Recently, the bright, shiny, freshly scrubbed look has been fashionable. To obtain this, a variety of abrasive materials is applied to the skin. These may be grains, buffing puffs, loofah pads, etc. These abrasive materials take off partially loosened stratum corneum cells, which in ordinary circumstances reduce reflectance of light, with greater dispersion and diffusion. The skin treated by these abrasives, when done properly, allows greater reflection of light over a relatively smoother surface. This imparts the freshly washed look of a more youthful, healthier skin. Second, these products produce mild trauma to the skin, which can induce temporarily increased blood flow as well as temporary edema. They have no long-lasting benefits. They do provide, however, a more reflective skin, which we associate with a younger look.

WRINKLE TREATMENTS

Applications claimed to reduce wrinkles are mostly hype. Collagen preparations currently on the market do not affect wrinkles in any permanent way. Some temporarily fill in creases analogous to putty filling in a crack in a wall, so that makeup placed over them will give the appearance of a less-deep wrinkle. Collagen molecules are too large to be absorbed through stratum corneum to produce any significant effect on sun damage and wrinkling.

The variety of techniques of facial exercises, taping one's skin up at night, and noon, are completely without basis. In fact, facial exercises should accentuate and cause more wrinkling, since certain wrinkles are due to muscle contraction. Increasing the number of times muscles contract can only worsen the condition.

The rubbing, slapping, and hot and cold water massage routines do provide a small temporary benefit. For probably two to three hours, more blood flows through the skin and, therefore, the pink tones show more. Similarly, edema can be produced in the skin by mild trauma, such as repeated slapping, which slightly reduces the visual impact of wrinkles. However, the effects are gone as soon as the traumatic edema has cleared. All of the special routines recommended by certain cosmetics companies seem to be pure hype, without substantial benefit. Possibly performing the ritualistic process helps the woman believe that she looks better, and believing that she looks better makes her feel better and thus behave in a manner more conducive to obtaining attention. In some women, therefore, the routines themselves have a positive effect. However, in our enlightened age, we know that everyone deserves the right to understand the mechanism of action. If they then accept the mechanism of action and wish to use certain routines with more expensive products, it is their choice.

SUMMARY

Cosmetics are an extremely important part of obtaining the greatest benefit for the patient.

The most important part of your involvement with makeup is adequate instruction of the patient. It is best to have someone in your office who truly understands makeup. This does not necessarily mean the person who makes herself up well, because she has been practicing on a single face for many years. Rather, choose someone who understands basic concepts of cosmetics and the variety of methods for application. If possible, train her or send her for a day or two of cosmetics training. The information she will impart to your patients will add to the excellent results you are providing through surgical methods.

Ideally, someone in your office should be well-versed in the use of cosmetics to assist patients. Since you have control over the situation, the patients will not be sold hundreds of dollars' worth of cosmetics that they do not need. If no one in your office has teaching ability, find a highly reputable professional who will recommend cosmetics. A number of professionals will teach women proper use of cosmetics and without selling them products. They often will tell the patients where the products can be obtained and sell only special products that cannot be readily obtained in nearby stores. A third choice is having a professional cosmetician in your office. However, you should obtain feedback from your patients to be sure that they are being instructed properly and sold those items that they need. There is a tendency in the cosmetics field to sell the patient as much as possible regardless of the patient's need. Cosmeticians learn a variety of sales techniques to persuade women to buy the greatest number of and the most expensive items. There are, however, many truly professional cosmeticians who sell only what a patient needs.

When a friend comments on the enhanced appearance of a patient, the effect produced by cosmetics is included in that evaluation. It is prudent for the physician to understand cosmetics and to have ready sources of referral for the patient. Poor application of cosmetics can detract from excellent surgical results. Proper individualized application of cosmetics enhances the benefits your surgery has provided.

18 / Epilation (Electrolysis)

EPILATION IS THE removal of unwanted hair, usually through an electrical means. The term implies an attempt to remove the hair permanently in contrast to manual epilation, i.e., plucking of hairs. Electrolysis, which commonly is misused interchangeably with epilation, produces permanent loss of hair by using direct current (galvanic current) to create sodium hydroxide at the hair papilla, thus chemically destroying the papilla.

In epilation the goal is to cause heat destruction of the root. Various high-frequency machines can be used for this purpose. A simple unit is the Birtcher hyfrecator set at the lowest current, with a small epilating needle attached. Bipolar current circuits are preferred because, theoretically, they discharge the current deeper in the tissue.

Though we have used a Cameron-Miller bipolar machine for many years, any number of high-frequency machines (Bovie, Valley Lab, etc.) with extremely low settings can produce epilation.

Professional electrologists favor certain machines that blend the amount of cutting and coagulating current. The claim for these machines is that they produce the quickest epilation with the least scarring. Certain machines may accomplish epilation a second or so faster than others, but a good operator seems to be able to work with most any machine. Although coagulation current is recommended for epilation, we have done it with coagulation or cutting currents and notice little difference in the final result.

PRINCIPLES

Important principles common to all epilation techniques are as follows:

Use of the thumb, forceps, and index finger inserting devices (Fig 18–1) described by DeFeo and Allyn[1] can speed epilation time by a factor of three. These must be custom made, but for any physician doing epilation, they are worth the cost. These simple devices make a usually slow task far more rewarding.

Pump the foot pedal. It should never be left depressed and continuously held down. The initial current that goes down the epilating needle comes off at the tip. As current is fed continuously to the needle, it will come off the sides as well as the tip of the needle. Since the goal is to produce a microburn deep in the dermis, destruction in the epidermis and papillary corium are unnecessary and are correlated with more noticeable scarring. The pedal should be touched, and as soon as the machine makes a noise or the light goes on, the foot rapidly should be removed. Three to five short bursts are far superior to one single burst of the same length of time.

Wear a magnifying lens. The plastic magnifying visors or a three-power set of reading glasses from the pharmacy are easiest for us to use.

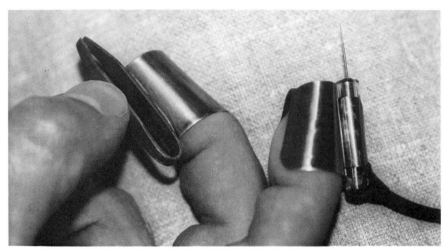

Fig 18–1.—DeFeo-Allyn epilating instruments.

TECHNIQUE

The epilating needle is inserted into a follicle and gently slid down the follicle until it reaches the bulb (Fig 18–2). This is perceived as a slight change in resistance felt in the fingertips, or it can be seen as a small indentation of the skin. If this feeling is not noticed, gently probe to make the needle go to the bulb or withdraw and start again. If you cannot be sure where the needle tip is, that hair should not be treated at that session, but at a future session.

With the tip of the epilating needle at the base of the follicle, short bursts of energy are delivered to the tip. With experience the operator learns the number of times to press the pedal of each type of machine. The epilating needle is removed from the follicle and the hair shaft grasped with smooth forceps or, preferably, with the DeFeo-Allyn device (Fig 18–3). If a sufficient amount of energy has been delivered to the root area, the hair will slide out of the follicle with little resistance. If there is any resistance, the epilating needle is reinserted and another set of short blasts of energy given. If the hair does not come out after the second burn, it is best to leave that hair for a future session. Repeated treatments to a single follicle at one session will result in visible scarring.

After treatment some antibacterial agent may be applied, although its value is unproved.

Within two or three days, small crusts will be seen in follicles. Sometimes this is charred surface tissue. Most often it is electrically coagulated tissue extruded from the follicle. The wearing of makeup is permitted two hours after treatment and probably is safe immediately after treatment. The patient is not restricted from engaging in routine activities.

Local anesthesia, particularly for the upper lip, is a welcome addition to epilation. For the upper lip, two infraorbital blocks are all that is necessary; for the chin itself, two mental blocks; and for lateral chin and neck, local infiltration may be used. Use of lidocaine with epinephrine is preferred because of its long duration.

A regrowth rate of 25%–50% is common. Since retreatment also has a 25%–

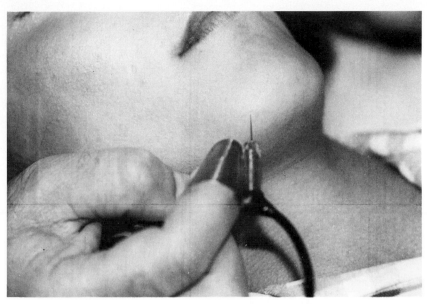

Fig 18–2.—Insertion of epilation needle.

50% regrowth rate, four to 12 sessions may be necessary to epilate an area completely. The hirsute woman undergoing epilation should plan for a one- to two-year program.

The number of hairs that can be done at a visit depends on the operator's skill, availability of a DeFeo-Allyn epilating device, the tolerance of the patient, and the distribution of hairs. Certainly, if you are treating the whole face, doing 100–200 hairs is not unreasonable from a physiologic point of view. However, to do 100 hairs on the upper lip would very likely result in scarring. It is best to space the epilation so that every second or third hair is done in a

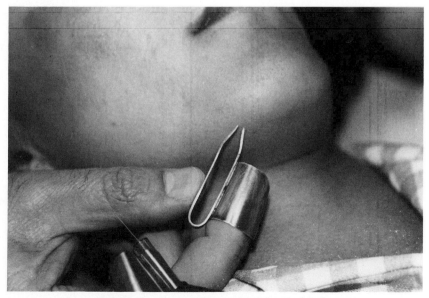

Fig 18–3.—Forceps to remove treated hair.

particular session, with plans to go back and remove the other hairs. This gives the tissue time to heal. Simultaneous microburns in adjacent follicles can result in a contiguous burn with an obvious scar.

Despite good machines, technique, and operators, some scars will occur in some patients. We have seen arms, backs, and chests totally epilated in sex-changed persons and have found it difficult to find a single scar. However, the same operator treating different patients has caused small, pit-like scars on the upper lip. Certainly, whether a scar occurs is due partly to the patient's inherent ability to respond to injury.

As of the time of writing this book, there are no machines that permanently eliminate hair without pain. Several other forms of energy have been explored, such as sound waves and microwaves, but none has been completely successful, yet.

Some recent work by Inaba and co-workers has shown that hairs that are plucked or destroyed by such procedures as completely cutting off the hair root and bulb from the underside will result in regeneration of new hairs.[2, 3] The scientific explanation is that new hairs derive from the isthmus of the follicle where the sebaceous duct enters the follicle. If this work is confirmed, it will go a long way to explain why the best people using the best machines still have high recurrence rates. The success of repeated epilation may mean that there is a limited number of hairs that the isthmus can produce.

Another simple form of permanent epilation is the battery-operated epilator. This produces direct current and heat at the tip. Again, the process is that of a microburn at the site of the hair root. There is little question that these machines are effective. The difficulty in using them is that the patient must learn to slide the probe to the bottom of the follicle and then endure the discomfort. Given the right patient, it is a successful method.

ELECTROLYSIS

True electrolysis is probably the oldest form of permanent epilation. Here, direct current from a battery source or by converting alternating line current into direct current is used.[4] The patient holds the positive electrode in the hand and the negative electrode is attached to the epilating needle. The procedure is the same as for regular epilation. The difference is that it takes 30 seconds to two minutes, depending on the diameter of the hair, to cause epilation of that hair. In electrolysis, the electrical current produces sodium hydroxide at the active tip to destroy tissue chemically. Although an electrical apparatus is used in electrolysis, it is a chemical destruction of the hair root compared with the heat destruction in high-frequency epilation. Usually, better control with superior cosmetic results can be obtained using true electrolysis. The problem of holding the needle still for approximately one minute per hair and the great number of hairs that need to be done render this form of treatment almost of historical nature. A few physicians and electrologists still practice this method.

SUMMARY

When permanent loss of hair is desired, epilation is the only reasonable approach. It seems that anything that works causes the patient pain, so patients should be told that machines that cause no pain do not destroy hair roots. Patients should be warned ahead of time that, depending on the amount of hair to be removed, they may need treatments every other week for one to two years. If this is acceptable, the modality is an excellent one in skilled hands.

Many dermatologists do not learn epilation, thinking that it is a dull, repetitive process that will bore them, but others find epilation a welcome part of practice. To be able to sit for 15–20 minutes doing a repetitive, mechanical process with immediate gratification can relax the mind while providing another service for their patients.

REFERENCES

1. DeFeo C.P., Allyn B.: Modified needle and forceps arrangement for epilating unit. *Arch. Dermatol.* 91:639, 1965.
2. Inaba M., McKinstry C.T., Umezawa F.: Regeneration of axillary hairs after plucking. *J. Dermatol. Surg.* 7:249-259, 1981.
3. Inaba M., Anthony J., McKinstry C.: Histologic study of the regeneration of axillary hair after removal with subcutaneous tissue shaver. *J. Invest. Dermatol.* 72:224-231, 1979.
4. Burdick K.H.: *Electrosurgical Apparatus and Their Application in Dermatology.* Springfield, Ill., Charles C Thomas, Publisher, 1966.

19 / Lipo-Suction

FOR MANY YEARS cosmetic surgeons have attempted to remove unwanted deposits of fat by excising it, shaving it out, or removing the skin and fat together. Dr. Richard Aronsohn of Los Angeles tried, unsuccessfully, to flatten the bulge adjacent to the nasolabial/meilolabial fold by inserting a long hypodermic needle through an incision in the vestibule of the nose to break up the fat in that area. His theory was that the traumatized fat would be resorbed and the deep scar tissue would flatten the area.

Japanese physicians invented a cutting device to control hyperhidrosis. When inserted beneath the axillary skin, this device trimmed off sweat glands from the deep portion of the skin. It also removed fat in a manner analogous to a subcutaneous lawn mower.

Italian physicians developed a cutting-crushing suction technique. The fat was cut or crushed and then sucked out. These instruments, however, cut too many blood vessels and resulted in hemorrhage.

French cosmetic surgeons, led by Dr. Yves-Gerard Illouz, improved the technique by using blunt-ended instruments to make tunnels in the fat from which dislodged fat then could be sucked out. These two steps and instruments were combined into one new approach. The same probe was hooked to a suction device that simultaneously broke down the fat and sucked out the loose fat globules. The French physicians used this safe, blunt-cannula technique for at least five years before it became appreciated by physicians around the world.

The value of injecting normal saline or hypertonic saline first is questionable. The French lay literature and reports appearing in the United States indicated that an injection of the saline first dissolved the fat that was to be sucked out. This step has been proven to be unnecessary and is no longer a part of the technique.

In the early 1980s, a number of American physicians traveled to France to observe the technique. Since that time, interest in the technique has mounted in the United States and other countries. The probes and cannulas, originally designed by the French physicians, have been redesigned to include better grips, cannulas with gentle curves for suction beneath the chin and around the curves of the trunk and extremities, removal of any sharp edges or points on the instruments, and the insertion of a window in the cannula handle so that the surgeon is able to see the quality of material being removed. It is important to know whether one is removing mostly fat, blood and fat, or mostly blood. Noel Robbins, a master instrument designer (Robbins Instruments, Inc., Chatham, N.J.), has worked in conjunction with Drs. Julius Newman and Richard Dolsky on the East Coast and Drs. Michael Elam, Fred Berkowitz, and Richard Aronsohn on the West Coast to provide a very effective set of cannulas for this technique.

THEORY OF ACTION

There are several theories as to why this technique is beneficial, and, as is common with a new technique, there is no strong evidence to support any of these theories. Time and repeated use with close follow-up will answer these questions in the future. One theory suggests that there is a specific and finite number of fat cells that do not divide. Once these are removed no other unspecified cells will differentiate and mature into fat cells. This theory is augmented by the suggestion that there are different types of fat cells and some compartments contain only "cellulite," which when removed, stays away forever. This theory has some faults in that it is well known that skin grafts can be defatted, and yet after several years in a new location, a great deal of subcutaneous fat is present on or under the graft. It is felt that some fat cells do arise from previously undifferentiated mesenchymal cells.

Another theory is that it is not the removal of the fat but the creation of a deep, subcutaneous scar that has more tensile strength and thus does not bulge as much as before the surgery. This fibrotic scar holds the tissues in and gives the appearance of less fat.

Some American physicians performing many lipo-suction techniques find that some of their patients have a greatly reduced appetite after the procedure and continue to lose weight because of decreased food intake. It is extremely hard to evaluate this type of report. However, the physicians are simply reporting what they see, and at this early stage of use and investigation, all reports must be considered and evaluated.

Nevertheless, there seems to be a definite improvement in the body contour, and it will be essential for all of us to observe how long this improvement lasts. In the meantime, whether it is loss of fat, temporary loss of fat, a subcutaneous scar formation, or some combination of the above, it is probably as close as we can come to understanding the theory at this time.

INDICATIONS FOR LIPO-SUCTION

Lipo-suction has value only for localized fat deposits. These are the same deposits that are the last to disappear in severe dieting or seem to never disappear even though the patient is at or below ideal weight. This is not a technique for generalized obesity. Some of the specific areas are the fat deposits beneath the chin and the nasolabial/meilolabial fold (Fig 19–1), the fat pads on the lateral hips and the so-called "love handles" on the flanks (Fig 19–2), the superior portions of the buttocks and the inferior portions of the buttocks (Fig 19–3), the mid-lower abdomen with the umbilicus at the center (Fig 19–4), and the localized fat deposits around the knees (Fig 19–5) and ankles (Fig 19–6).

EQUIPMENT

We use the equipment made by Robbins Instruments, Inc. (Chatham, N.J.), with a pump vacuum of greater than 29 in. of mercury. The cannulas are hollow and the blunt end has a crosscut configuration so that the cannula will "lock onto" the fat in front of it and not be deflected into areas of less resistance. Cannula lengths are 7 and 8.5 in. for facial work and 10 and 13 in. for body work. Some physicians find the cannulas with a slight curve more effective for the submental area and for going around the curves in the abdomen,

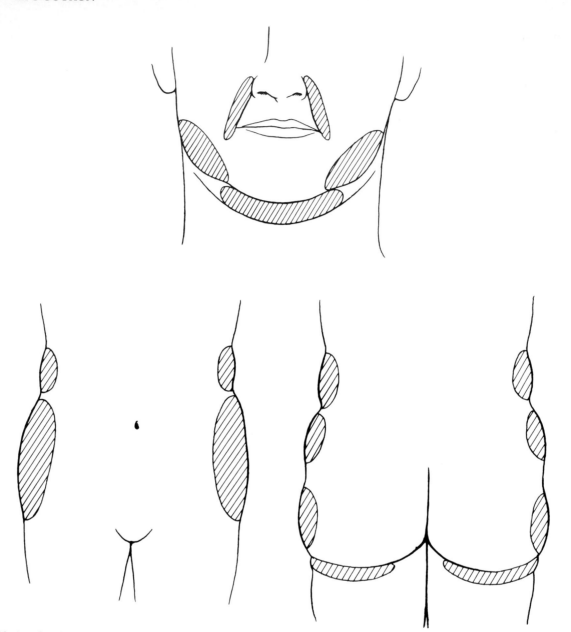

Fig 19–1.—(*Top*) The areas of the face and submental region which respond to lipo-suction. The nasolabial area is accessed through a small incision inside the lateral wall of the nose just posterior to the attachment of the ala. The jowls and submental region are accessed through a small incision just posterior to the posterior inferior edge of the mentum.

Fig 19–2.—(*Bottom left*) The lateral hips and the "love handles" on the flanks are accessed through small incisions just lateral and posterior to each of those fat deposits.

Fig 19–3.—(*Bottom right*) The posterior view of the "love handles," lateral thighs, and lateral and inferior buttocks. A small incision just at the lateral edge of the gluteal cleft provides good access for the lateral buttocks and the inferior buttocks area.

thighs, and buttocks areas. For beginning work with lipo-suction, we suggest cannulas that are 4, 6, and 8 mm in diameter. The 6 and 8 mm diameter cannulas can be used for abdomen, hips, thighs, knees, and ankles. The 4 and 6 mm diameter cannulas can be used for the submental fat pad. The 4 mm cannula or the 3 mm cannulas, which are now in production, can be used for the nasolabial/meilolabial fold. As the popularity of the technique grows, specific sets for facial or body work will be developed and available. It is our feeling that the Robbins instruments will become standard because of the development of the window into the design which allows for continuous monitoring of what is being aspirated.

TECHNIQUE

First, an incision through the skin just slightly longer than the diameter of cannula is used to gain entrance to the desired area of fat. The location of this incision is placed where it will show the least: in the folds of the umbilicus or the suprapubic ridge for abdominal work, in the submental crease for the submental fat pad, and just inferior to the gluteal fold for work on the buttocks.

Second, a pair of blunt-nose scissors is inserted perpendicular to the skin to deepen the incision into the fat pocket. The cannula is inserted and the surgeon uses his other hand to grab the fat and pull it up into a roll in front of

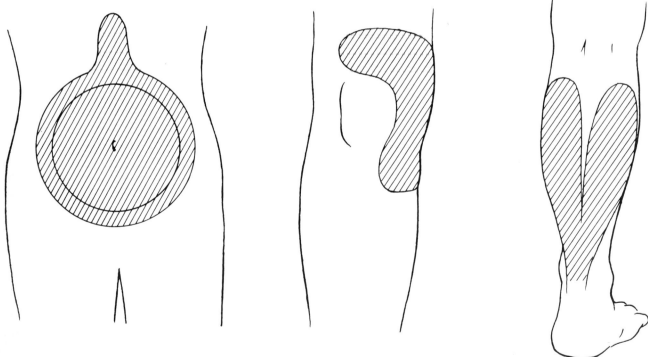
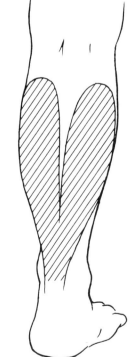

Fig 19–4.—*(Left)* The mid-lower abdomen with an extension on some people toward xiphoid area responds very well to lipo-suction and is accessed through almost invisible small incisions in the umbilicus.

Fig 19–5.—*(Center)* The medial edge of the knee and the inferior medial area of the quadriceps often has an unsightly fat area which responds to suction through a small incision at the medial edge of the knee.

Fig 19–6.—*(Right)* The inferior one-half of the leg and around the posterior surfaces of the ankle respond to lipo-suction through a small incision usually on the medial surface of the lower leg near the Achilles tendon area.

and around the cannula as the cannula is pushed forward. The first step is to push the cannula up into the rolled fat held in the surgeon's opposite hand to break up the fat. The cannula is advanced towards the surgeon's other hand so that the surgeon always knows the depth of the cannula and where the tip is located. This adds safety and also improves the results of the technique. With experience, the surgeon learns how to adjust the level of his probe to gain desired effects.

When used on the body, this technique requires a considerable amount of physical effort. The cannula is worked back and forth, advancing it further and further until it has reached the desired area. The tunnels should be made deep in the fat so as to avoid damage to the dermal plexus, which is between the dermis and the fat. Once the desired length of tunnel has been created, the suction is turned on. The cannula is worked back and forth as it is slowly withdrawn. Fat tinged with a small amount of blood is seen through the window of the cannula. If a great deal of blood is seen in the window, the cannula should be withdrawn or be repositioned. The presence of blood means that the aspiration part of the cannula is against a blood vessel. Although there is some blood loss, it is surprising how little blood is aspirated in lipo-suction.

The cannula is then withdrawn to the original starting point in the deep fat and directed in a different radius or direction. The process is repeated until the desired number of tunnels have been created in the fat and aspirated.

It is always wise to be conservative in fat removal and to be sure to leave an adequate layer of fat on the inferior surface of the skin flap. Taking fat too close to the skin or taking too much fat can lead to irregular adherence of the skin to the underlying tissue, thus creating dimpling, ridging, and ruffling of the skin surface. One can always return at a later date for a second procedure to remove more fat if necessary. One of the theories is that the goal is to remove enough fat so that the tunnels will collapse inward thus obliterating the tunnel effect but also leaving a more pleasing external contour.

Sometimes suction drains are left in the area if it appears that there is an excessive amount of serosanguineous exudate. These negative suction drains can be the Davol type, or more simply, intercath arrangements attached to blood-drawing vacuum tubes. If the latter is used, the patient needs to be instructed on how to change the suction tubes.

TAPING

Once the area has been completely sucked, it is covered with a tape. Presently, many cosmetic surgeons use a product developed in France, which we can compare to Elastoplast available in the United States. However, we suspect that more efficient ways of taping will be available soon.

It is important to put pressure on the areas sucked so that the fat will collapse into the tunnels, hemorrhage will be controlled, and the integument will be supported after it has been injured so extensively.

The submental area is best taped with strips of tape starting on either side of the midline of the anterior neck. It is not proper to use one long piece of tape that runs from one cheek under the chin to the other cheek, because it will cause wrinkling and ruffling of the skin. The taping should be done meticulously and care should be taken to be certain that the first layer is absolutely smooth on the skin.

It is appropriate to follow other physicians' techniques. However, we suspect that many alternative methods in taping will be reported. The use of 3 × 3 in. gauze squares, covered with any of several good tapes available in the United States, may be perfectly adequate for the submental area.

On the hips, abdomen, knees, and other areas, longer strips of tape can be used. Again, the first layers must be laid down meticulously and pressed evenly onto the skin. As is always true, tapes should not be placed circumferentially on any extremity. Women undergoing abdominal or hip lipo-suction can use a firm girdle in place of the tape.

The tapes are left on for seven to ten days. It is a good idea to ask the patient to sit in the tub, use one of the available medical tape removers or vegetable oil as adjuncts in order to remove the tape.

ANESTHESIA

Most cosmetic surgeons use general anesthesia when doing this procedure. However, there are several French physicians who have done the procedure with local anesthesia for many years. We see no reason why small areas cannot be done with local anesthesia, and large areas done one section at a time under local anesthesia to avoid the cost and risk of general anesthesia and the need for an expensive hospital operating room.

Using 0.5% Xylocaine with epinephrine 1:200,000, the patient can tolerate up to 100 ml before toxic levels are reached. Adding hyaluronidase, 1 cc per 30 ml of Xylocaine, permits better spread of the anesthesia through the tissues, thus giving wider anesthesia with a small volume.

For specific areas on the face, such as the submental fat pad, regional nerve blocks can be applied by injecting the mental nerve as it exits the mandible on the chin and by blocking the cervical sensory branches that emerge at the medial edge of the sternocleidomastoid muscle.

Hips, knees, and the thighs are usually done with the wide local infiltration technique.

RESULTS

Thus far, this technique is very popular in France and is gaining popularity in the United States. We do not have the benefit of long-term follow-up of a significant number of patients to make any comments about the final outcome or the longevity of the results. This is a new technique and must be approached carefully by all physicians. No warranties or guaranties should be implied. We are not satisfied with any of the long-term data, but feel that this technique merits use and development. With an open and fair contract with the patient, there is no reason why individuals who suffer with unwanted fat in certain areas should not benefit from the technique as long as it proves to be safe.

The results are not readily apparent. Patients are advised that when the tapes are first removed they will be disappointed and their disappointment will last for weeks or months. There can be generalized or localized ecchymoses, the skin will often look irregular with the tunnels appearing more ecchymotic or depressed than the surrounding areas. It takes several months for the fat to even out and some of the ruffling of the skin to smooth out. This generally happens some six to eight weeks after surgery, and then the patients become happier with their profile. Some patients have discomfort for several weeks, but most patients are completely ambulatory immediately after the surgery and are limited only a little in their quiet activities. Vigorous physical activity is discouraged until the patient is pain free.

Most important is the surgical judgment. To accomplish successful lipo-suction, the skin over the area of fat to be removed must have sufficient tone and elasticity so that it will tighten after the desired fat is removed. Excessively aged, sun damaged, or inelastic, redundant skin may have a worse cosmetic appearance following lipo-suction. Patients who are fairly young and have localized fat deposits with normal elastic skin overlying those deposits are the best candidates for the procedure.

MEDICAL INDICATIONS

Lipo-suction will remove large lipomas—8–10 cm or larger—through a 1 cm incision. Previously, an 8–10 cm incision, with the equally as long resultant scar, would be needed for removal of these lesions. Similarly, patients with multiple moderate-size lipomas can have them all removed through very small incisions.

Medically-induced buffalo humps secondary to long-term treatment with corticosteroids also can be removed through a small incision on the posterior neck area.

Pseudogynecomastia is treatable with small incisions at the edge of the areola or inferior to the breast mass itself. This is an embarrassing problem for some men, and this is the best treatment to date for that problem. This can be accomplished fairly easily under local anesthesia, but appropriate hormone tests should be done to rule out a true gynecomastia. Lipo-suction is not currently recommended for reduction of breast size in females. It is best to use the standard surgical mammary reduction approaches for the female breast.

COMPLICATIONS

Ecchymoses and soreness in the area is expected in everyone. With abdominal lipo-suction, the well-motivated patients say they feel as though they had done too many sit-ups. The less-motivated patient may complain of uncomfortable, subcutaneous pain for many days. Some patients who have relatively small areas treated with lipo-suction, such as the "love handles," may be operated on Friday and back to work Monday. Other patients with much larger areas treated need to stay off work for seven to ten days.

So far, bleeding in the postoperative period has not been a significant problem. A small amount of ooze can be expected in the drains or a more significant ecchymoses if drains are not used.

Loss of skin sensation has been reported and is much the same as any surgical undermining. This generally returns to normal within two to three months after the surgery.

If excess fat has been removed from the undersurface of the skin, scar tissue forms in that area and can cause puckers, dimples, or irregular contours. This is particularly annoying in the submental region or areas that show during some activities. As the wounds gradually remodel over the first six to eighteen months, most of these irregularities smooth out.

A troughing or ridged effect can be seen if the lipo-suction was excessive along the tunnels. Here, the skin surface appears indented in a linear fashion. This can also occur if the cannula was passed from an area with a thick fat pad into one with very little fat and too much fat was sucked from the undersurface of the skin. These types of errors in technique lessen as the physician becomes more skilled and experienced.

The goal of most lipo-suction is body contouring, and much of the clothing hides areas where the actual suction took place. Again, it is important to emphasize to the patient that immediately after surgery they will not see much improvement. The improvement comes with time as the wound remodels and the scar formation takes place.

We have not heard of any examples of the skin sloughing. Sloughing is expected to be highly unlikely with the new, blunt cannulas that have been developed in the United States. Neither have we heard of motor nerve damage, but this, too, can be expected in a small percent of the cases until more physicians become skilled and experienced.

FLUID REQUIREMENTS

The amount of fat removed when large areas are being treated must be recorded. If 500 ml of fat and fluid are removed, the patient is usually replaced with 500 ml of an albumin solution or a similar blood expander. A greater than 500 ml replacement is made on the basis of 1 ml of volume expander to 1 ml of fluid removed. There are some red blood cells lost, and therefore, the patients may need to take supplemental iron.

In order to limit red cell loss, some physicians load the patient with 2 liters of intravenous fluids prior to the surgery. Because of this dilution, there are fewer actual red cells lost. The combination of the hemodilution with this preloading of intravenous fluids, plus the true red cell loss may cause a significant drop in the hematocrit.

Replacement with transfused whole blood or packed cells has not been common or even reported with this technique. It is not known how much fat and fluid can be safely removed. Most surgeons feel it is prudent to remove less than 1,500 ml in total. That amount is replaced at the time of surgery with plasma expanders or normal saline.

CONCLUSION

Lipo-suction is an exciting new modality and will provide the cosmetic surgeon with yet another tool for body sculpting. Lipo-suction in the submental area appears to be a quicker, faster method than the current tedious techniques of scalpel or scissor excision used to contour the submandibular area. The unwanted fat bulges which appear resistant to dieting and exercise in the abdomen, hips, and ankles seem to respond well to this method. Large lipomas, buffalo humps, and pseudogynecomastia are also easily treated through the small inconspicuous incisions.

Although some physicians have been using the method for five years, good long-term follow-up is not yet available in the literature. Lipo-suction should be considered a new technique requiring specific training both in courses and at the operating table with experienced physicians. It is probably best to remove too little fat than too much. Secondary touch-up procedures can always be done six to nine months later when the scar formation and edema resolution are complete. The fact that this can be done in an office setting with local anesthesia makes it particularly attractive to the office-based cosmetic surgeon.

Index